9.95
1.88

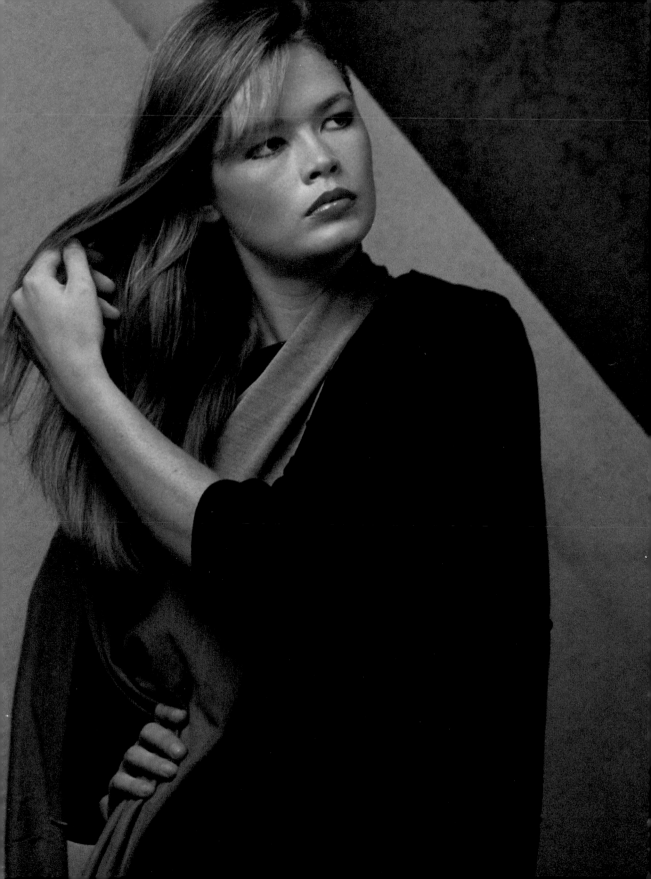

COLOR YOUR HAIR

COLOR YOUR HAIR

by
Peter Waters

A Lucy-Caroll Book

An Owl Book
Holt, Rinehart and Winston
New York

$\overline{6}$

■

Published in the United States by Holt, Rinehart
and Winston, 383 Madison Avenue, New York,
New York 10017.

Library of Congress Catalog Card Number: **83-83102**

ISBN: 0-03-070504-5

First American Edition

Created and produced by:
Lucy-Caroll Limited
228 Gerrard Street East,
Toronto, Ontario
Canada M5A 2E8

Designer: Rod Della-Vedova
Photographer: Greg Lawson
Editor: Shelley Tanaka
All hair by the group at Jason Kearns Inc.

Printed in the United States of America

10 9 8 7 6 5 4 3 2 1

Warning: Every care has been taken in the preparation of this book to detail the necessary precautions required when applying hair color. However, the author and his publishers assume no liability whatsoever for any loss or damage resulting from the application of the processes and products described herein.

$\overline{7}$

■

For Mum and Dad
for all the things you are
and G.S. – my inspiration

As you can imagine, a book of this kind involves a great many people. I cannot list them all, but I would like to thank: Jason Kearns for his encouragement and friendship; my colleagues at his salon for all their help; Judith Finlayson for a magnificent writing job and Shelley Tanaka for being a great editor; Greg Lawson for his superb photograpy; Rod Della-Vedova for his inspired design and art direction; Lucienne and Gordon for their beautiful make-up and all the models who gave so generously of their time. Lucinda Vardey and Carolyn Brunton, who battled with me and for me, and without whom this book would never have happened. Finally, my thanks to Melinda for all her love and encouragement.

Peter Waters
January 1984

CONTENTS

CONTENTS

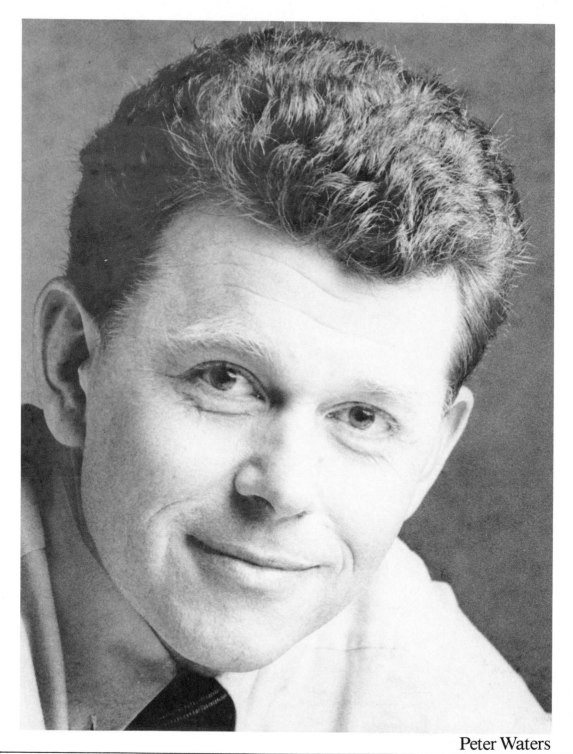

Peter Waters

C O L O R   Y O U R   H A I R

INTRODUCTION

My most vivid memory of my first day in hairdressing is that of walking through the door of the salon and being overcome by the pungent aroma of permanent waving lotion. Then, once I was safely beyond the threshold, I was told that I'd have to change my name.

"We already have a Peter," I was informed. "What's your middle name?"

"Leonard," I answered without thinking. So Leonard I was for the first few years of my career.

It was hardly an auspicious beginning. But over the past twenty years my career has had its ups as well as its downs, and has ultimately brought me a great deal of satisfaction. If there's one message I want to convey, it's that I sincerely love what I do. I've written this book because I want to share some of the excitement I find in my work with you.

One of the people I met that first fateful day was the owner of the salon, a bald-headed man named Leslie Green. It's safe to say that without him I wouldn't be where I am today. He talked me into learning about color, and for the next six years he steered me on the course that led to my career as a color technician.

When I first became an apprentice, hair color was just beginning to emerge from the dark ages. Most clients had either a permanent wave, a tint, a bleach or highlights. We were on the threshold of being able to achieve the living, natural colors we have today.

As much as I complain about those products of bygone days, in the grand scheme of things we had a lot to be thankful for. Hair may have looked a bit unnatural, but at least the products were safe. This had not always been the case. Horror stories about the effects of ancient dyes still circulate today. Often these concoctions were both unreliable and dangerous. We can only imagine what must have happened to some of the women in ancient Rome who bleached and crimped their own less-than-perfect tresses because they wanted to have long golden locks. No wonder wigs have been so much a part of our fashion history.

It took the Golden Age of Hollywood, the fabulous 1930's, to change society's attitude toward hair coloring. Stars such as Mae West, Jean Harlow and Carole Lombard reigned supreme as glamour girls. Moreover, all freely admitted that their hair color was artificial. A crucial part of their dazzling image was their own creation.

By the time Lana Turner, Marilyn Monroe, Rita Hayworth and Jane Russell were at their peak, some twenty years later, the public took for granted that their hair was colored. Although her fans knew that Marilyn Monroe was a natural light brown, no one perceived her to be anything other than a stunningly beautiful blonde. Eventually it became more than just acceptable to color your hair. When Rita Hayworth, already a star as a redhead, changed her hair to blonde, she was making a definite fashion statement.

Hollywood's influence went hand in hand with improvements in the safety and effectiveness of hair coloring. Prior to 1930, henna was the only hair coloring agent available commercially. In order to color hair blonde, it was necessary to bleach it with a mixture of henna and hydrogen peroxide, the strength and stability of which could not be controlled. Not only were the results unpredictable, but the colors were harsh and unnatural.

By the late 1950's, however, the technology had advanced to such a point that companies such as Clairol, Revlon and L'Oréal had developed hair coloring products that were both safe and easy to use. Within a few years, amateurs could purchase the same semipermanent and permanent hair colors previously reserved for professionals. And purchase them they did, spurred on by massive promotion campaigns such as Clairol's "Does She or Doesn't She?" With one of the most successful advertising campaigns in history, Clairol contributed to the revolution that was brewing in the hair coloring business.

About the same time that I was living my professional life as Leonard, everybody began to talk about a new name in hairdressing – Vidal Sassoon. In the salon where I worked, we were still doing roller sets and backcombing hair, but the newspapers were showing pictures of innovative geometric cuts. My boss, Leslie Green, had helped to train Sassoon early on in his career. He urged me to go and take a look for myself.

So on my day off, I went to Sassoon's and stood outside the salon to watch the haircuts come out. The street was like a zoo. Everybody had come to see what all the fuss was about. It was so exciting that, then and there, I decided that my ambition was to work for Vidal Sassoon.

And thirteen years later, that's exactly what I did. The emergence of my own most creative work is directly linked to that experience, because I had the great fortune to work with the people at Sassoon's who launched the revolution in hair color as we know it today.

But I also have a very practical purpose in mind. I want to provide you with a technical understanding of what hair color involves. Coloring your hair is not that complicated if you know how to do it. If you don't, you can make some dreadful mistakes.

Certainly there are many excellent color technicians around the world. However, some of the most horrendous mistakes are made by hair-dressers themselves. A surprising number know very little about hair color, and they have made little or no effort to learn. And yet they consider themselves qualified to color your hair.

It is one of the strange paradoxes in hairdressing that while we have made many advances in how we cut and style hair, it is only in the past six years that there has been any real attempt to improve the hair coloring techniques of the last two decades. These new ideas are certainly beginning to filter through — both in the salon and in the development of home products — but not as quickly as some of us would wish. My feeling is that if I can provide you, the client, with the appropriate information, you in turn can spur your hairdresser on to greater knowledge.

Once you become familiar with the various hair coloring techniques outlined in this book, you should decide which one is right for you by asking yourself what you want from your hair color. If, for instance, you want a very complex color effect, you must be prepared to invest more time and money than is necessary if you are happy to have your hair highlighted once every six months. In other words, before you can choose from the variety of alternatives that this book presents, you must decide how much time, money and effort you are willing to devote to your hair.

Moreover, before you set out to color your hair, you must be aware that all of the techniques included here are only recommended if you have not colored your hair before. **If you already have a permanent color on your hair, if you have bleached it or if you have a permanent wave, you should not attempt to color your hair at home.** You must see a qualified hairdresser.

There is also a product available today which is technically called a progressive dye. This is a permanent coloring product that is worked into gray hair over a period of days to eventually change it to a shade of brown. These products are also completely incompatible with any permanent wave, temporary, semipermanent or permanent hair color, bleach, toner or highlights. If you have used one of these progressive dyes, you should not attempt to color your hair. The results could be disastrous. You may end up with bright metallic pink or green hair.

I also don't think that it's a good idea to color your hair until you are at least fifteen or sixteen years old. Leaving the hair free of chemical treatments until that time will give it the opportunity to grow strong and healthy.

I believe that you will find this book particularly useful because my knowledge of hair coloring does not stop at the salon. I make a point of keeping myself informed about what is available for the home market, not only because I'm interested, but because I'm often asked to correct mistakes that people have made using these products.

And finally we've come to the most important consideration of all — safety. For although hair coloring products are safer and more effective than ever, it is still vitally important that they be used with great care. Basically, this means that before *each* application of any hair coloring product you must test yourself to make certain that you are not allergic to that product (see page 41).

Although each set of instructions outlined in this book reminds you to take a preliminary sensitivity test, I want to emphasize just how important this simple procedure is. Don't be lulled into a false sense of security because the odds are against you developing an allergic reaction to any of the products. At best, allergic reactions are unpleasant. At worst, they can be terrifying.

This said, I hope you will enjoy this book and that it will start you thinking about adventures in coloring you hair.

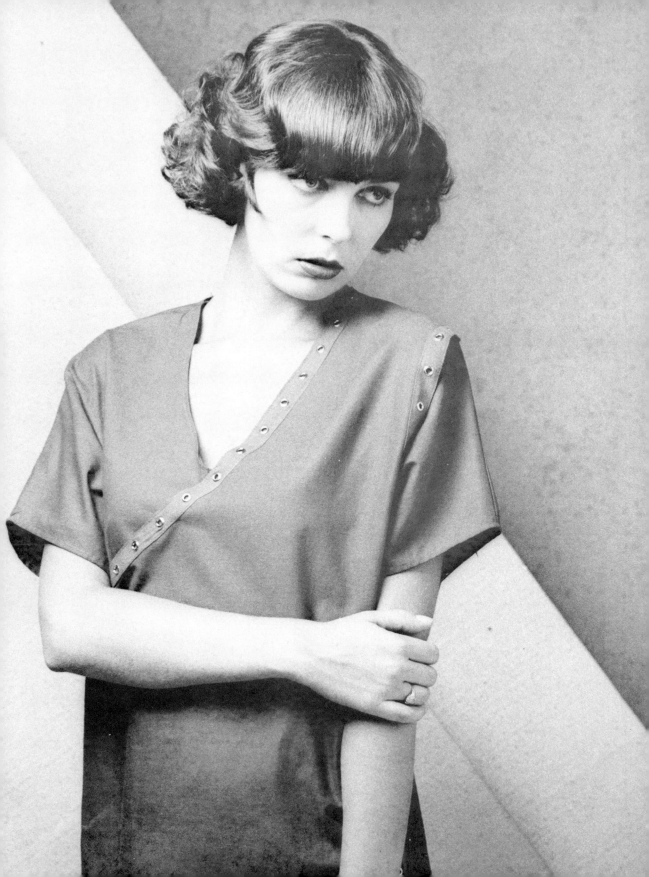

The Nature of Color

THE NATURE OF COLOR

THE PRIMARY COLORS; SECONDARY COLORS; THE PRISM; TERTIARY COLORS; COLOR WHEEL; COMPLEMENTARY COLORS. HOW COLOR RELATES TO HAIR.

I first learned how to color hair at the L'Oréal school in London. The course lasted one week, and on subsequent weeks I attended similar sessions organized by Clairol and Wella. It was 1965, and all I had to know was how to choose a color and how to apply it. So after three weeks I had apparently learned all I needed to know to be able to color a client's hair with a degree of confidence.

They must have taught me well, because I don't remember any disasters. My point is, however, that although I learned how to use the manufacturers' particular products, no one taught me anything about the nature of color and how it relates to hair. If there is only one thing I hope to impress upon you by the time you finish reading this book, this is it: **You must understand the nature of color and how it relates to hair — your own hair in particular — if you want to change your hair color successfully.**

We've all seen blondes — a friend calls them "jungle blondes" — whose hair is brassy yellow or greenish looking. Or redheads whose medium copper blonde tresses turn out, on closer inspection, to be pink at the temples. These mistakes and many others result from not knowing how colors interact. They can be avoided by learning the general principles of light and color as they relate to hair.

White light, which is the light that surrounds us, reflects all the colors of the spectrum as it travels through the atmosphere. It is the opposite of darkness, which is the total absorption of color, reflecting no light at all.

This concept can be difficult to grasp, unless you can actually see it by using a prism (see Figure 1). When white light hits one side of the prism, the light rays bend to reveal that the white light we see is actually composed of seven colors: red, orange, yellow, green, blue, violet and indigo. These are known as the *spectral colors*. (Of the seven spectral colors, only indigo has little relevance to hair coloring. Indigo has such a short wavelength it has no large role to play in our understanding of color as it relates to hair. Moreover, it has no complementary color, the importance of which I'll explain shortly.)

The way we perceive color depends upon how the light rays bend. As you can see by the illustration of the prism, the ray that bends the least has the longest wave length. This gives us the color red.

Figure 1

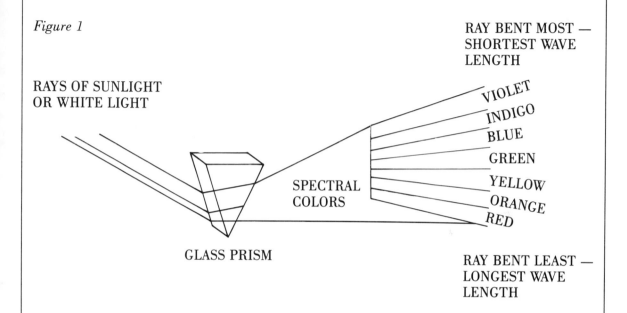

RAYS OF SUNLIGHT
OR WHITE LIGHT

RAY BENT MOST —
SHORTEST WAVE
LENGTH

VIOLET
INDIGO
BLUE
GREEN
YELLOW
ORANGE
RED

SPECTRAL
COLORS

GLASS PRISM

RAY BENT LEAST —
LONGEST WAVE
LENGTH

PRIMARY COLORS

The most important of the spectral colors are known as the *primary colors*. They are red, blue and yellow and they form the basis for all other colors. Just as musical notes lay the groundwork for musical compositions, so are complex colors built upon combinations of primary colors.

SECONDARY COLORS

The secondary colors are orange, green and violet. They are formed when two primary colors are mixed:

    red + yellow = orange
    yellow + blue = green
    blue + red = violet

Every natural hair color and every artificial hair coloring product is a blending of primary and secondary colors.

TERTIARY COLORS

When we mix two or three secondary colors, we achieve different shades of brown. For example:

$$green + violet + orange = dark\ brown$$
$$orange + green = medium\ brown$$
$$orange + violet = light\ brown$$
$$green + violet = ash\ brown$$

These brown colors are known as *tertiary colors* and can be broken down into one, two or three blends of the primary and secondary colors.

THE COLOR WHEEL

Figure 2

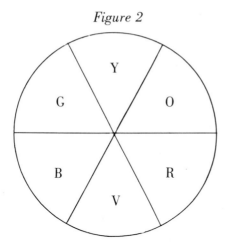

PRIMARY COLORS   SECONDARY COLORS

YELLOW   ORANGE
RED   VIOLET
BLUE   GREEN

The color wheel may be the best way to explain how we mix colors (see Figure 2). As you can see, orange, which is a combination of red and yellow, lies between them on the color wheel. Violet is a combination of red and blue, and green results when blue and yellow are mixed.

COMPLEMENTARY COLORS

Notice that violet appears opposite yellow on the color wheel. Red is opposite green and blue is opposite orange. These are known as *complementary colors*, because if you place red beside green, blue beside orange, or yellow beside violet, each color will appear at its clearest and brightest. When complentary colors appear side by side, neither color detracts from the other.

However, when you *mix* complementary colors together, they neutralize each other. I can vividly remember one evening when I was having dinner with a friend who was wearing a royal blue blouse. Our table was bathed in a soft orange light and I noticed that her blouse, which I knew to be blue in natural light, appeared to be black. This was easily explained. In the restaurant the orange light was shining on a solid blue background, through which no light could pass. All the orange light was absorbed by its complementary color, and black appeared to be the result.

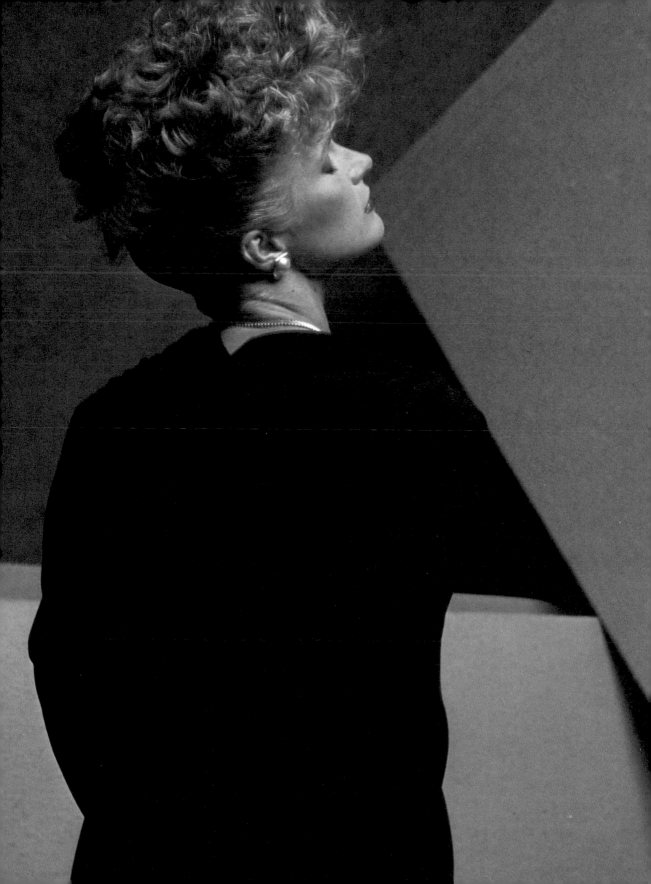

You might find it interesting to pair colors that are not complementary. If you place a piece of blue paper next to a piece of red paper, you will notice that each color takes on something of the other. The red looks slightly bluish and vice versa and neither color seems quite as clear as before.

When colors that are not complementary are paired, the intensity of the original colors is diminished because each color is mixed with some of the other. Basically, they clash because they arrive at the eye, simultaneously, like two noisy children demanding mother's attention simultaneously.

You will remember from the diagram of the prism (Figure 1) that each color has its own wavelength, with red being the longest and violet the shortest. The colors that clash (red with orange, yellow with green, blue with violet) have wavelengths of approximately the same length. On the other hand, the complementary colors, red and green, blue and orange, yellow and violet, vary greatly in wavelengths.

To further enhance your understanding of the laws of color, try one final experiment. Get a small set of crayons and mix any two or three secondary colors (orange, green and violet) together. You'll find that you have varying shades of brown, ranging from light to dark. Add green to all the existing shades. The browns will darken and take on ashen tones. Make the same basic shades of light, medium and dark brown again. Then add orange and notice that the color immediately becomes warmer, brighter and lighter. Suddenly you're seeing colors that are similar to natural hair color. Both natural hair colors and hair coloring solutions are made up of combinations of these primary and secondary colors.

HOW COLOR RELATES TO HAIR

Since we can't actually see colors such as blue, green or violet in hair, it's natural to ask how we *know* they are really there. Think of the prism again, and remember that light is composed of seven colors, but none of them is visible to the naked eye.

Similarly, we don't see the pigments in the color of hair until the structure of the hair is actually broken down. The best way to expose these tiny molecules of color inside the hair shaft is by bleaching. Even so, we still only see the warm colors — red, orange, yellow and pale yellow — because the other colors are not visible to the naked eye.

Chapter 7 is devoted to the subject of bleaching as it relates to coloring your hair. But at this point, I would like to summarize the process because it helps to explain the nature of color in relation to hair.

Bleach is a mixture of ammonia and hydrogen peroxide. When these two elements are combined, a mild heat results which causes the mixture to expand (oxidation). This softens the outside of the hair (cuticle), causing it to open up. The mixture can then penetrate the inside of the hair shaft.

Depending on the natural color of the hair, the process varies slightly. Black hair, for example, has pigment in all the primary and secondary colors. It consists of approximately 70 percent red and green pigment, 25 percent orange and blue pigment and 5 percent yellow and violet pigment. As the bleach penetrates the inside of the hair (the cortex) these various pigments begin to break down, some more quickly than others.

First the process removes the green pigment and the hair turns red. Then the red and the blue pigments are removed at about the same pace, revealing orange. The violet pigment (a mixture of red and blue) is stubborn but eventually most of it comes out. Gold is the result. It is only when the violet pigment is finally removed, that we see the pale yellow that forms the basis for many spectacular platinum blondes.

The same process occurs when you bleach red and blonde hair, only some of the steps are removed. When bleach is applied to red hair, for instance, orange-gold will be the first color to reveal itself. When blonde hair is bleached, it will first turn gold, then yellow-gold and finally pale yellow.

My clients often ask how hair can be different colors if every head of hair contains all six colors. The answer is that the proportion of the pigments is different. Light brown hair contains mainly orange and blue pigments, with much less but almost equal amounts of red, green, yellow and violet. Light blonde hair is chock-full of yellow and violet pigments, but has meager amounts of orange and blue pigments and even less red and green.

It may surprise you to know that there is such a thing as hair without pigment. Very simply white hair is hair that is colorless. Color is produced in an organ at the root of the hair (papilla) by melanin, the same natural chemical of the body that colors our skin. Melanin, however, can't reproduce itself. Consequently, as more and more melanin glands die, the hair grows in colorless.

You'll be interested to know — and this is important when you set out to color your hair — that there is no such thing as gray hair. "Gray" hair is actually an optical illusion created when white hair mixes in with hair that is naturally brown or black.

When no one color predominates in a head of hair, the overall effect is of mousiness. Because the complementary pigments are present in equal amounts, they neutralize each other.

When I was teaching at Vidal Sassoon in London, I realized that some of my students were having difficulty understanding this concept of mousy hair. So I devised an experiment to prove my point. I created mousy hair from hair that was not mousy to begin with.

Beginning with a head of very light natural blonde hair, I painted tiny dots all over the head, using all six primary and secondary colors, in exactly the same proportion. They neutralized each other and the hair deepened in color. But it was a definite shade of mouse. Unfortunately, most of us have hair that tends to be mousy, which helps to explain why we're so easily tempted to color our hair.

Now that you understand the fundamentals of color and how they relate to hair, you can apply this knowledge to your own hair. In the following chapter, I will show you how to identify the natural color of your hair and how to select the color change that is not only most flattering to your appearance, but also compatible with your needs and general lifestyle.

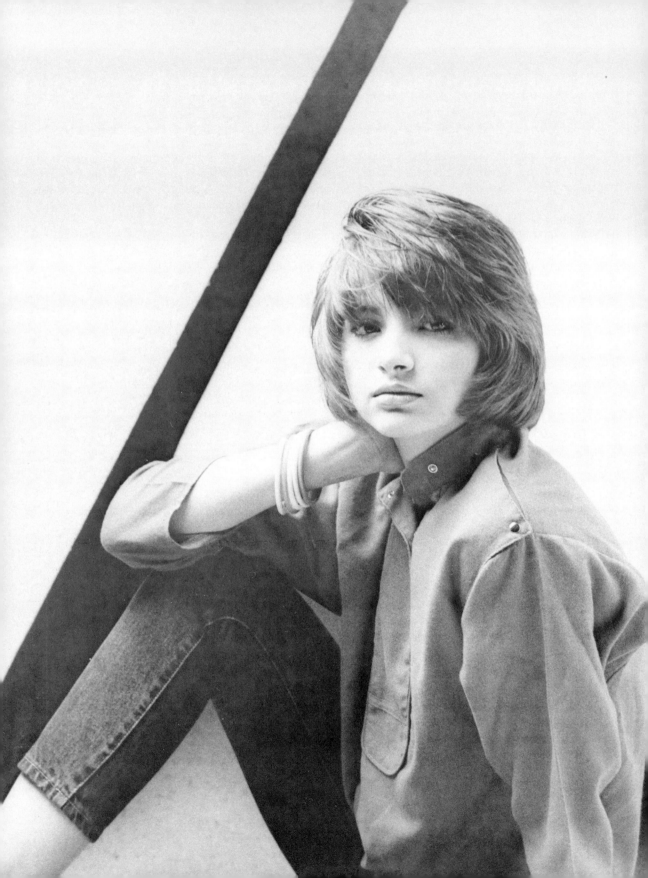

YOUR NATURAL COLOR

YOUR NATURAL COLOR

THE COLOR CHART —
IT'S PURPOSE AND HOW IT WORKS;
SPECIAL NOTES ON RED HAIR.

When I began learning about color in England, it was 1965. I was taught the basics in only five days by each manufacturer, but in those days this was thought to be enough, even for professionals.

Today, manufacturers of hair-coloring products offer advanced color courses — basically because we now have a fairly wide body of knowledge about color as a science and how it relates to hair. I teach some of these courses myself and I'm able to do so because over the years I've increased my own knowledge by studying books on painting and color. I've also refined my hair-coloring technique through simple trial and error.

Color technicians starting out today have access to extensive information which their predecessors had to learn on their own. But at the same time they have a far greater range of products which they must fully understand in order to offer their clients first-rate service. Certainly, men and women working in the field today can have much more fun with color than those of us who started out years ago.

Even so, I learned a lot in those dark ages that still stands me in good stead. For instance, in those brief courses which I took almost twenty years ago, I was introduced, to an invaluable chart system that simplifies the essentials of hair coloring. My own version is the color chart that appears on page 26.

THE PURPOSE OF THE COLOR CHART

The color chart is designed to do three things:

1. It enables you to pinpoint your natural color quickly and accurately.

2. It allows you to predict the result when the color of your choice is applied to your natural hair color. (Remember, since every head contains all the pigments in varying proportions, the same product will produce a different result on every person.)

3. If the color chart indicates that applying the color of your choice to your hair will not result in the color you want, it will reveal how to adjust your choice in order to achieve the desired result. If it is not possible to achieve this result, given your natural color, the chart will make this clear. At this point you must either choose another color or see a professional color technician.

HOW THE CHART WORKS

Before you can change the color of your hair, you must determine what its natural color is. The column on the left of the color chart lists the basic natural or neutral color types. Hairdressers call these *color depths* or levels.

Each color depth has been assigned a number which appears on the chart. They range from black (number 1) to extra light blonde (number 9). This is the range within which you will be able to experiment at home. Professional color technicians have about four more levels at their disposal. Many of us have hair that is basically one color flecked with another — usually ash, gold, orange or red. These appear horizontally on the chart as *tones*. They must also be considered when you are planning to color your hair.

For example, if you have light brown hair that is tinged with gold, you must locate that particular color combination on the chart. Light brown appears on the level of color depths at number 4. Now, since you also know that your hair contains gold, look across the tones to the column headed "gold." Let your eye travel down that column until it is parallel with number 4. This space contains the description "light golden brown." That is the color of your hair.

The basic colors that appear on my chart also appear on the charts put out by manufacturers of hair coloring products. These charts can also help you to determine exactly what your natural color is.

In order to determine your natural color using the guides produced by the manufacturers of hair-coloring products, cut several strands of your hair from the nape of your neck (about twenty strands should be sufficient). Take this hair sample along with this book to your local drugstore, where you will find the manufacturers' coloring guides — rows of colored hair swatches that indicate what color the various products will produce. Pick any one. At this stage all you want to do is to find the swatch that is the same color as your hair sample.

The color swatches in the manufacturer's sample will be grouped under several headings very similar to the ones I have used in my chart. First look under the basic natural color section. If your natural hair color has no dominant tone, you may find a perfect match there. The manufacturer's color guide may, for instance, describe this color as "dark golden blonde." Locate that description on my color chart and asterisk it. It is a description of your own natural hair color.

COLOR CHART

COLOR DEPTH		TONES			
NUMBER	NATURAL/ NEUTRAL	ASH	GOLD	ORANGE (COPPER)	TRUE RED
9	extra light blonde	extra light ash blonde	extra light golden blonde	extra light copper blonde	extra light pinkish blonde
8	very light blonde	very light ash blonde	very light golden blonde	very light copper blonde	strawberry blonde
7	light blonde	light ash beige blonde	light golden blonde	light copper blonde	light reddish blonde
6	medium blonde	medium ash blonde	medium golden beige blonde	medium copper blonde	flame red blonde
5	dark blonde	dark ash blonde	dark golden blonde	dark copper blonde	dark reddish blonde
4	light brown	light ash brown	light golden brown	light golden chestnut brown	light warm chestnut brown
3	medium brown	medium ash brown	medium golden blonde	medium golden chestnut brown	auburn brown
2	dark brown	dark ash brown	dark golden brown	dark golden chestnut brown	burgundy brown
1	black	blue black	*	*	*

*There are no tones of black other than blue black.

It is more likely, however, that you will not find a basic hair color that matches your own hair sample perfectly. This only means that in addition to being a basic color, your hair has a tone of a different color — most likely ash, gold, orange or red.

If, for instance, your hair has gold tones, locate the color swatches that are grouped under the manufacturer's heading "gold." Try to match your hair sample to one of the swatches here. If you find a perfect match, read the description of the color on the manufacturer's sample. *That* is your natural color. Find the same color on my chart and asterisk it. This is an important step. Otherwise, you might forget how to describe your natural hair color in terms of the chart.

Warning: The artificial lighting that you find in most stores will affect the color of both the hair swatches on the manufacturers' charts and the color of your own hair sample. If you are unsure about whether the artificial light is affecting the color, ask a shop clerk for advice or take the swatches and your hair sample out into the natural daylight (check with the clerk first, so there won't be any misunderstandings). Or you can find a store that provides facilities that allow a comparison to be made in natural light. A surprising number of stores do offer this service.

Red Hair

If you have red hair, you will notice that you are not represented on the color chart from levels one to nine. This is because red hair is a tone of a color. Red hair can be as light as a light strawberry blonde, or as dark as a burgundy brown. Red hair can also have orange tones. For instance, medium copper blonde is actually medium blonde hair with orange tones. Understanding these differences is crucial to redheads who are coloring their hair. Before coloring their hair, redheads, like everyone else, have to match a sample of their own hair with the swatches provided by manufacturers.

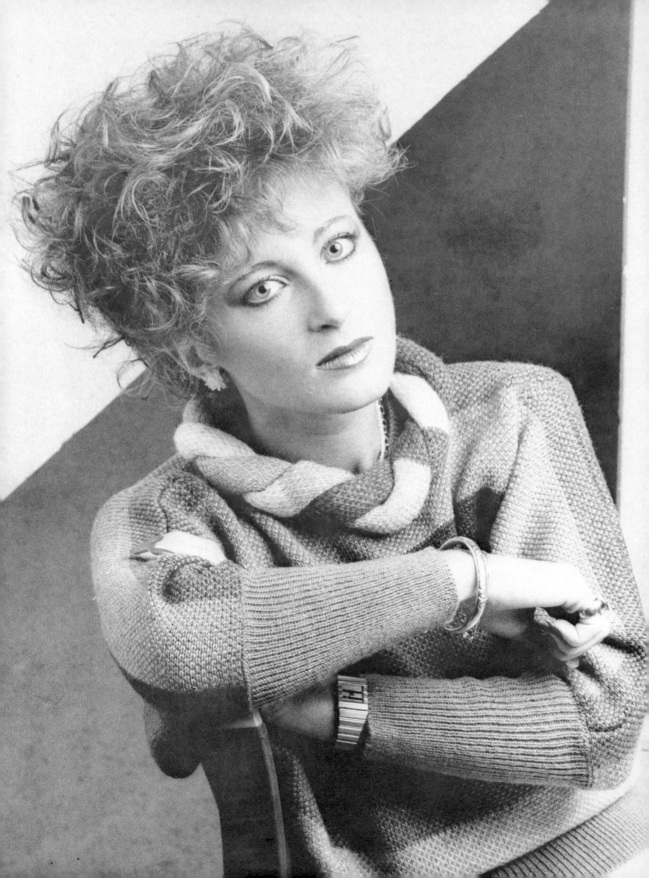

CHOOSING YOUR NEW HAIR COLOR

CHOOSING YOUR NEW HAIR COLOR

RULES FOR CHOOSING A NEW HAIR COLOR; GOING DARKER, GOING LIGHTER AND BRIGHTER; THE SEXINESS OF BLONDE; THE ROMANCE OF RED; THE CLASSIC BROWNS; SOFTENING THE EFFECTS OF AGE: GRAY HAIR.

Now comes the fun part — deciding what color you want your hair to become. For me, this is far and away the most exciting part of the business. Over the years, my own observations have convinced me that the most dramatic results I've ever seen in hairdressing salons have been created by color.

Nowadays some hair-coloring procedures are more complicated than the ones I learned in 1965.

For instance, now it's not unusual to use color to emphasize shape and cut – something that no one even dreamed of twenty years ago. The result can be subtle, such as highlights in bobbed hair that is all one length. As the hair swings through the wind, the color flows with it. All you see is beautifully healthy and alive hair that doesn't look colored.

At the other extreme are some of the punk looks we see today. The hair is cut into extreme shapes and the dramatic use of color increases the provocation. The result is a look that's so aggressive that it's impossible to ignore. But it's not really that different from the first look. In the end we have two heads of hair which must be noticed — the first because it's so beautiful, the second because it's so strong.

So here you are, about to set out on the exciting adventure of coloring your hair. The first step is to determine what your natural hair color is (see Chapter 2). Then, using the color chart, you can decide what your potential color choices are by following these basic rules:

1. If you are coloring your hair at home, **you should never move more than two levels up or down on the color chart.** If you want to change your hair color by more than two levels, see your hairdresser.

2. **Do not change the tone of your hair.** If you wish to change the natural tone of your hair, you would be wise to see a professional. If your hair has gold highlights, for example, you will achieve the best results by choosing a new hair color that is also in the gold tone group. If you have naturally mousy hair (hair with no predominant tone) you can add any tone you want.

3. **Your new hair color should complement your skin tones.** If you have pink skin tones, you should not use a color with red tones. The similarity in the tones of the skin and the hair will make the face and the hair blend together and appear as something of a blur. Similarly, people with golden beige skin tones should steer away from colors with gold tones. Although you should exercise discretion, the orange tones *can* go with either skin tone. Let your own cautious eye be the judge.

Let's assume that you have put your hair through all the tests outlined in Chapter 2 and have decided that your hair is light brown, with no predominant tone. On the chart, light brown is at level 4. Using our first basic rule, this means that any of the colors within two levels up or down (levels 2 through 6) are well suited to the natural color of your hair. And because your hair is mousy, you can also choose any of the tones that appear within levels 2 to 6. Light warm chestnut brown will add red tones. Medium copper blonde will lighten and add orange; dark golden brown will darken and add gold.

Which of these colors is best for you? Be careful. All will work with your hair to produce a perfectly natural result. However, some will flatter you more.

Do you have pink skin tones? If so, don't use a color with red tones. A color with orange, gold or ash tones (e.g. light golden brown, light golden chestnut brown or light ash brown) is a better choice. Not only will the orange, ash or gold tones soften your skin tone, but the pink in your skin will show the hair color to better effect.

If, on the other hand, your complexion is pale golden beige, a red tone will give your skin needed warmth.

GOING DARKER

If you are under thirty-five, dark hair can be very effective because it can emphasize your eyes and facial features in a very flattering way. But if you are over thirty-five, dark hair has a tendency to look hard — basically because it calls attention to the lines that are beginning to show on your face.

These lines are nature's way of softening your features as you age. White hair contributes to the same effect. By coloring your hair darker at this stage of life, you are going against nature. The softening of your features doesn't mix with the high drama of the color. It can have a jarring effect.

Nevertheless, there is a situation in which coloring the hair darker is very advantageous. If you have very thin hair, the last thing you want to do is call attention to it. The darker the hair, the less it reflects the light. Thus, by making your hair a level darker than it is naturally, you can create the optical illusion of thicker hair.

Warning: Do not follow this theory through to its logical conclusion. Making the hair black will not give it the desired appearance of abundance. It's more likely that the result will be a hard, unnatural color.

DRAMATIC BLACK

Black is one of the most dramatic of all color changes. If you are under thirty-five, black can be used to dramatize the shape of a hair cut. Black, however, is so dramatic that it's easy for someone to get bored with it. If that's the case, it must be either stripped (which will damage the condition of the hair) or cut out. The effects can be fairly devastating. Another word of warning: Black tints stain the skin and will show more than any other color. So you must be very careful when using them.

The first time I ever tinted a client's hair, she was going to black. I wasn't aware that black tint would stain the skin. As you can imagine, I was also extremely nervous. I did succeed in coloring her hair, but I also colored her arms, her neck, and liberal parts of her face. She was the tea lady in the salon in which I worked, and whenever I see her she still laughs about it. It was 1963 — maybe by now she's forgiven me.

GOING LIGHTER AND GOING BRIGHTER

"Lighter" and "brighter" are two concepts you should understand before setting out to change the color of your hair. Going lighter means exactly what it says. If, for instance, your hair is light brown (level 4) and you wish to become dark blonde (level 5) you would be going lighter. Similarly, if your hair is light brown and you wish to become a dark ash blonde (dark blonde with an ash tone), the end result would be lighter but not brighter than your light brown hair.

However, if your hair is light brown and you wish to become a dark golden blonde (dark blonde with a gold tone) your hair will appear both lighter and brighter. This is because you have added a warm tone which has brightness in it. Those warm tones are gold, red and orange. Adding them will brighten your hair. An ash or neutral color, on the other hand, absorbs light and consequently will lighten your hair without brightening it.

Rule of Thumb: The warm tones (orange, red or gold) will increase the brightness of a color. The ash tones will reduce the brightness of a color.

This experiment with crayons will show you what I mean. Mix equal parts of orange and violet together to create brown. Then mix twice as much violet with the orange. The light brown will appear much darker. But if you mix twice as much orange with the violet, the color will be *much* brighter than the second example and somewhat brighter than the first. That's what happens in hair color. The ash tones contain violet which absorbs the light and makes the hair color appear darker.

THE SEXINESS OF BLONDE

Redheads are fiery, and brunettes may smolder, but if there's one hair color that symbolizes sexiness, it's blonde. Marilyn Monroe was the quintessential blonde, the woman whom gentlemen apparently preferred, and her influence inspired thousands of women to take the color plunge. Unfortunately, not all of them were successful. This book will explain and tell you how to avoid the same mistakes.

As you can see from the chart, technically speaking, blondes begin at a level 5, which is only one level ligher than light brown. However, when most people think of blonde they think of hair that is light blonde — a level 7 or lighter. So when we talk about blonde, we will talk in terms of being blonde, as the general public perceives it to be. That's all the colors that appear on the chart from level 7 (light blonde) to level 9 (extra light blonde).

Let us assume that you are, technically speaking, a level 5, dark blonde, even though I am sure you think of yourself as light brown. Your hair has ash tones. Therefore, your natural hair color is dark ash blonde.

Since there are so many shades of blonde, you might do well to thumb through a few magazines, ripping out photographs and making notes of the colors your particularly like. But remember to consider your own natural hair tone (ash) and your own skin tones. If your skin has a pink tone, steer clear of the red tone blondes (e.g. flame red blonde, level 6). They are better suited to blondes with golden beige complexions. This will leave you with the foolproof options of the light ash colors.

Look through the photographs and choose the picture with the shade of light ash that you prefer. Match this picture up with the manufacturer's swatches which you have used to determine the natural color of your hair. Let us assume that your desired hair color is light ash beige blonde. Different manufacturers will have different names for that color. Let's say they call it "Fantasy Dawn." The name sounds great, but it doesn't tell you a thing about the color. But under the name will be a description of what the color in the bottle actually is. It will verify that this is, indeed, light ash beige blonde.

To achieve this effect you will have to use a *lighter* color in the same group. The procedure is simple. Because you want to lighten your hair by two levels (from a 5 to a 7) you would choose a product that is two levels lighter than the target color. To lighten your natural hair color (level 5) to a light ash beige blonde (level 7), you will use an extra light ash blonde tint (level 9). Your natural color, dark ash blonde, consists mainly of yellow and violet pigments with only minute traces of orange and blue. Therefore, as the extra light ash blonde tint lightens your hair, the violet pigments in the tint will neutralize the unwanted yellow in your own hair. Thus you will be able to achieve your target color, light ash beige blonde.

But suppose your hair is naturally darker than dark blonde. Herein lies the explanation for one of the most common errors people make trying to go blonde. If, for example, your natural color is light brown (level 4) and you apply the same tint (extra light ash blonde) your hair will end up brassy. Light brown hair contains a lot more orange and blue pigment than dark ash blonde hair. The violet in the tint will not be strong enough to neutralize the gold deposits in the hair as it becomes lighter. Your hair will end up looking like a medium golden beige blonde. Thus the "brassy" look.

Rule of Thumb: If you want to become a "true blonde" your natural color should be no darker than dark blonde (level 5).

If your hair is light brown, and you want to be a light ash beige blonde, you can do one of three things:

1. **Choose another target color** — one that is within two levels of your natural color.

2. **See a professional colorist**. A highlifting tint, only available in salons, could accomplish the desired result. Salons have colors that will accomplish more than those available to the general public. The manufacturers of products for the home market must build in greater safeguards because they have to assume that the people who are using them know nothing about coloring hair. In essence, they're trying to save you from yourself, to prevent you from ending up with green hair when what you wanted was a nice golden blonde.

3. **Bleach your hair**. But this is something I don't recommend, though highlighting with bleach might be an alternative.

A word of warning about golden blondes. These are very tricky, even if gold tones are already in the hair. In that case, gold on gold intensifies and the results can be too strong. If you are a golden blonde and want to go lighter, you should stick to a neutral color or a color with ash tones, even though the result you want to achieve is a definite golden blonde.

If you do not have gold tones in your hair, changing your hair color to a golden blonde can be equally tricky. A pure golden blonde is such a precise color that you only have to be slightly off target to end up with a color that's too bright and brassy. On the other hand, you can err on the side of caution and end up with hair that's mousy.

Given this problem, I would recommend that at home, you should only try to create a true golden blonde effect (level 7 or 8) if your natural color is light or medium blonde (levels 6 to 8). The gold pigment in the hair is already exposed and, therefore, the subtlety of adding a gold color is just enough to swing the balance away from a neutral color to gold. The results should be dazzling.

When you don't want to color your hair all over with one color, then a subtle way of changing the color is by highlighting. If your natural hair is a level 5 or lighter, then you can use blonde or bleach highlights (Chapters 7 and 8).

THE ROMANCE OF RED

I'm probably biased, because my own hair is red, a shade of dark copper blonde, but red is my favorite hair color. It's also a color with great versatility. Even nature seems to be attracted to redheads, since she gave us henna, a plant which we can use to color hair red.

What do we mean when we talk about red hair? A good question. Everyone has a completely different idea of what red hair is. For the purposes of description, I have broken it down into three categories: 1. gold 2. orange 3. true reds

Red hair is further complicated by the fact that it can run the gamut from very light blonde (level 8) to dark brown (level 2) in terms of color depth.

Because red occurs in all levels but one (level 1, black) color depth is virtually irrelevant. Technically, anyone can become a redhead. However, again you should consider your natural hair and skin tones. It is especially important to consider skin tones with reds because there are gold reds, orange reds and pink reds. The gold reds complement and soften pinkish complexions, whereas the pink reds perform a similar service for golden beige complexions. The orange reds, if properly chosen, can go with either.

When going red, consider the pigments that your natural color contains. For instance, if your hair is medium or dark brown, the strongest pigments in your hair are red (see Chapter 2). So if you wanted to become red, you should use a color that appears under the red column (auburn brown, burgundy brown). If your hair is blonde, the general rule is that the medium blondes have orange pigment, making medium copper blonde a good target color and the lightest have gold or what appears to be pink. In this case, light strawberry blonde would be a good choice if you wanted to add red.

Rule of Thumb: Be cautious when adding red, if you're going lighter. You may get more than you bargained for.

If you are going lighter and you want to add red, this is one situation where it would be wise to select a color that's one level higher than your target. So, for instance, if your hair is a naturally dark blonde (level 5) and you want to become a medium copper blonde (level 6, orange) I would advise that that's the color you apply. You're only using a product that's one level lighter, but it will deposit enough of the orange pigment to brighten your hair dramatically and create the desired effect.

If you want to color your hair red you can also consider adding red highlights. For example, when red hair gets dull, often after you reach the age of thirty-five, it can come alive again by adding red highlights (see Chapter 8).

A note on strawberry blonde: This appears on the chart at level 8, very light blonde. Any light blonde (level 7 to 9) can become a strawberry blonde, including those with ash, gold, orange or red tones in their hair, because it has pinkish-beige overtones, not gold. It is also one of the colors that goes with most skin tones. Almost anyone can wear it, as long as their skin tones are not **too** pink.

A note on burgundy brown: This is the darkest red, appearing at level 2 on the chart.

Because the power of the color is, in effect, in its depth (like a bottle of burgundy wine it is dark and rich) it loses its effectiveness when it's too light. Therefore a burgundy tone is most effective on either medium or dark brown hair (levels 2 and 3).

A note on golden chestnut browns: These appear under the oranges in the lower brown range, levels 3 and 4. The truest chestnut — medium gold chestnut brown — will give a deep rich golden brown effect. It is a color that flatters many age groups, as it can soften a fading dark brown. It can really enhance dull brown hair that appears lifeless. On younger women it helps to deepen their hair color, giving greater emphasis to eyes and bone structure.

THE CLASSIC BROWNS

There are four basic levels of brown hair, from black (level 1) to light brown (level 4). If you have naturally medium or light brown hair, and you're under thirty-five, you may want to darken it a shade or two to produce a more dramatic effect. You may even want to go black. Or you may want to improve on your brown color if your hair is mousy, or if you have some percentage of gray. If you don't want red in your hair, your options are the ash or neutral tones. You can also add more interest to brown hair by adding gold, orange or red highlights (see Chapter 8), or by adding henna, a natural dye that will give your hair a red or rich brown color.

SOFTENING THE EFFECTS OF AGE: GRAY HAIR

You'll remember from Chapter 2 that there is actually no such thing as gray hair, that it results from an optical illusion created when white hair blends with hair that still contains color. So gray hair is, by definition at least, two tones — natural brown or black mixed with white.

Because white hair has no pigment, it accepts any color at face value. Thus, if light copper blonde (level 7) was applied to white hair, the result would be a vivid orange, since the predominant pigment in light copper blonde is orange. Where white hair exists, therefore, we must add another color to the artificial color we are using — one which contains more of the basic pigments found in the neutral color at the same level. In this case that would be light blonde (level 7) and those pigments would be yellow and violet.

Rule of Thumb: Because white hair contains no pigment, we must make sure that the color we apply to white hair has an equal balance of pigments. So we mix equal amounts of neutral color at the same level with the desired color.

In order to determine the color that should be applied to gray hair to achieve the desired result, we must ask, as always:

1. What is the natural color? If you take a few strands from the darkest area, you will be able to determine this with the aid of the color chart at a drugstore. Use your natural color. Don't take the gray into consideration.

2. What color do you want to be?

3. What is your skin tone?

When a client comes to me with gray hair, she usually wants to return to the color she used to be. More often than not, this is a mistake, for the same reason why women should not go darker after age thirty-five. White hair is nature's way of softening the effects of aging on our faces. Thus, what used to be our natural color can tend to look hard when we're older.

The quantity of white hair and its location on the head are important in determining what color you are going to use and whether to use more than one color. For example, if the white hair is only around the face, and the rest of the hair is looking a bit dull, you may want to get rid of the white and liven up the rest while you're at it. In this case, you would have to purchase two different colors. For instance, if you decided that your natural hair color was dark blonde (level 5), you could apply a neutral dark blonde color to your white hair. But because color on color goes darker, you would have to use a medium blonde (level 6) on the rest of the head. You could also use a medium golden beige blonde on your natural color, which would give your hair a definite highlight.

One hundred Percent White
If you are completely white, you will likely only need one color, but because white hair has no pigment you must stick to the neutral tones. Moreover, because the change from white hair to no white hair is a dramatic one, you should keep it in the light blonde shades. They correspond most closely to your natural level.

Fifty Percent White
In this case the white hair will have a definite lightening effect on the whole head. So it's safer for you to go lighter than darker. Stay within the medium blonde to light brown range (levels 4 to 6). These colors are most likely to flatter you because you will be going along with the natural tendency of hair to lighten as you get older.

Twenty Percent White
You should use a color that is only one level lighter or darker than your natural color. Or if your hair is only 20 percent white and you wish to remove some but not all of the gray, brown highlights can be added to remove some of the gray and blend in with your natural hair color. Because this highlighting procedure is not as easy as it might appear, it is something that should only be done in a hair salon.

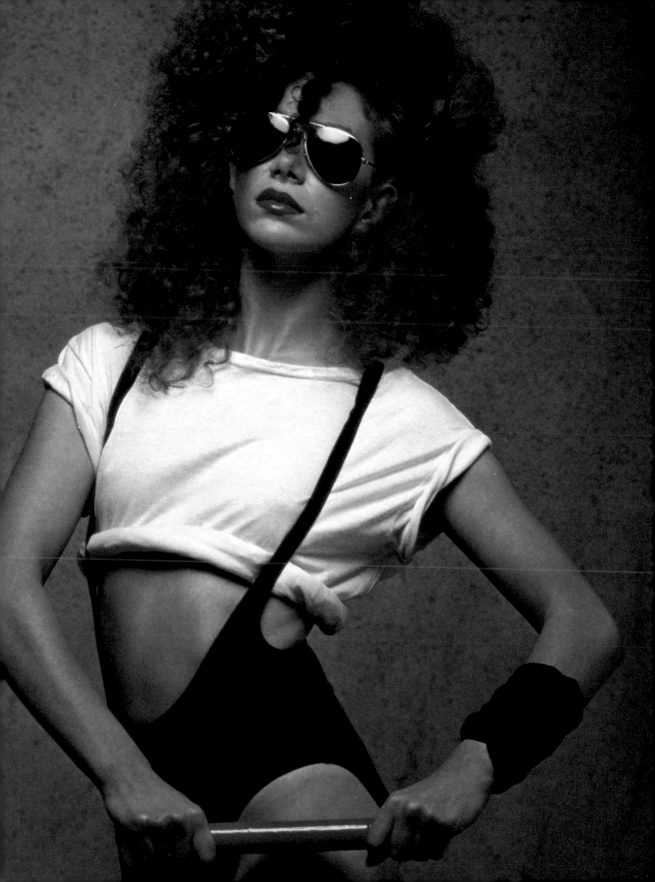

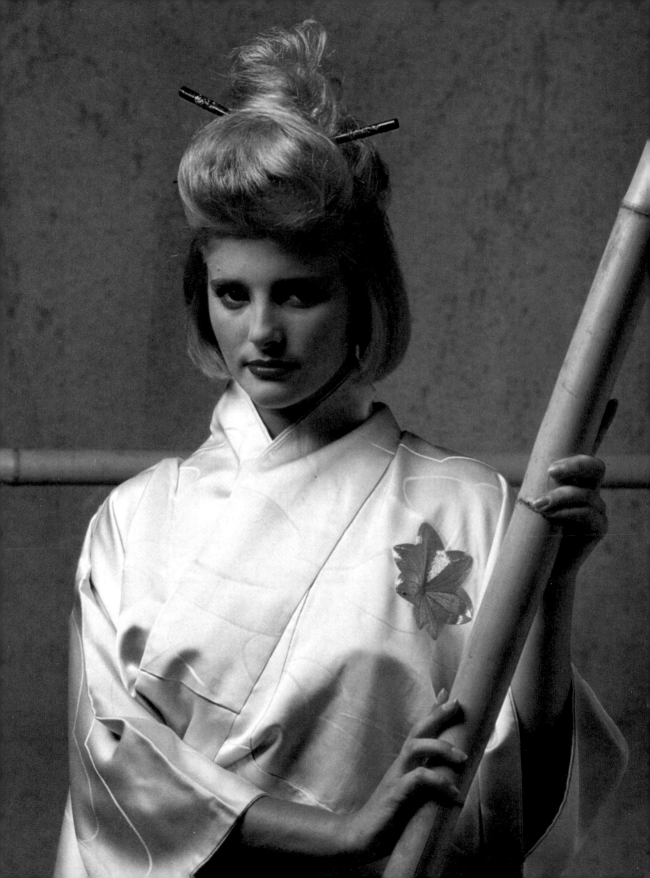

WHAT ARE YOUR PRODUCT OPTIONS?

WHAT ARE YOUR PRODUCT OPTIONS?

HOW TO GIVE A SENSITIVITY TEST; WHAT TO DO IF YOU HAVE BECOME ALLERGIC TO TINTS; HOW TO DO A STRAND TEST; WHAT IS THE RIGHT PRODUCT FOR YOU — TEMPORARY COLOR, SEMIPERMANENT COLOR, PERMANENT COLOR, BLEACH, HIGHLIGHTS OR HENNA?

Since I started working as a colorist, probably the greatest single change I've seen in the business has been in the range of products available for coloring hair. Today, there's so much more to choose from in terms of color and quality that it's easy to wonder how we ever managed before. This is true for the home market as well as for professional products.

Needless to say, this is partly due to the response by manufacturers to public demand. Quite simply, more and more people are having fun with hair color. A world-wide survey conducted in 1955 revealed that of the women who visited hair salons, 70 percent went to have some form of color applied to their hair. In 1980 another world-wide survey showed that only 35 percent of the women who went to a salon did so to have their hair colored. But over that period of time the sales of home hair coloring products increased by 50 percent. This suggests that a vast number of people who used to have their hair colored in a salon are now doing it at home.

Moreover, in the past five years in major cities such as London, New York, Milan, Paris, Munich, Toronto and Los Angeles, there has been a dramatic increase in the number of people who are coloring their hair, both at home and in a salon. More people are having their hair colored today than at any other time in history.

To some extent this is linked to the graying of the baby boom. The children born after the Second World War were part of the largest population explosion in history. These men and women are now in their thirties, and many have started to go gray. Their sheer numbers have had a definite effect on hair color sales.

So, too, the influence of the Sixties. Those were the days when "unisex" salons first made an appearance and men began to go to women's hairdressers because they didn't want to have "barbered" hair. I can remember when they would come in at the end of the day so that no one could see them. But gradually men became comfortable with the idea that they could have the same things done to their hair as women. Permanents were the most obvious result. Then coloring began to become popular too.

The downside of this interest in hair color is that people are doing it themselves and often they're making dreadful mistakes. The classic case is the woman who wants to go blonde, so she picks up the box that contains the color she wants to be. Instead of a nice natural ash blonde, she ends up with bright yellow hair, for reasons we've previously discussed.

Anyone who frequents stores where hair coloring products are sold can watch these horror stories in the making. Because store clerks are not qualified color technicians, their knowledge is, at best, rudimentary. Nevertheless, people insist on asking them for advice and the store clerks are inclined to give it.

One of the most common bits of bad advice that store clerks are likely to give concerns the difference between a "rinse," or semipermanent hair color, and a permanent hair color. Time and time again, clients will come to me with color on their hair which, they were told, would wash out after six shampoos. In fact, they were sold a permanent hair color which will not wash out. It stays in until it grows out. This can take anywhere from three months to two years, depending upon the length of the hair.

One more word of warning. The latest product to hit the market will likely be very prominently displayed in the store where you decide to buy your hair color. You must be very careful when you're buying hair coloring products. Make sure that you're not succumbing to a great sales pitch and advertising. These are often not the products you need.

Moreover, if you've already colored your hair and you're changing to another product, you must go back to basics. Take a swatch of your natural hair and relate it to the manufacturer's colors swatches, just as you did the first time you colored your hair. Also do a strand test at home. The product might not be identical — even if they are made by the same manufacturer and even if the colors have the same name.

Rule of Thumb: Before using any hair coloring product there are two things you must always do: Before **each application**, give yourself a sensitivity test and do a strand test. For the sake of convenience, both can be done at the same time, forty-eight hours prior to using the product.

HOW TO GIVE A SENSITIVITY TEST

1. Clear an area about the size of a dime behind one ear.

2. Put on rubber gloves.

3. Take a capful of the product you will be using (if using bleach or permanent color you will have to mix up an appropriate amount according to the manufacturer's instructions) and dab some of it onto that area.

4. Wait 48 hours. If you are among the 0.1 percent of the population that is allergic to the tint, you will notice the development of a slight irritation. If this happens, wash it off immediately and do *not* color your hair. I'm not being overly cautious. The allergic reaction is very unpleasant — some people puff up like balloons — and it can be very painful.

What To Do If You Have Been Coloring Your Hair and Suddenly Become Allergic to the Tint

1. Stop tinting your hair.

2. Check with your doctor and explain what happened.

3. No one wants to walk around with their regrowth showing, and there are some possible alternatives:

a) You might be able to cover your regrowth with a semipermanent rinse. However, you may have some difficulty matching the regrowth to your permanent color, particularly if it is lighter than your natural color. In that case, you will have to darken your whole head with a semipermanent color. (There is still a possibility that you'll be allergic to the semipermanent color. So you must do a sensitivity test and await the results before applying the color.)

b) Some hairdressers may recommend tinted highlights because the color does not touch the scalp (highlights always start at least 1/8 inch away from the scalp). But I believe that this remains a risk, and I personally don't advise it.

c) After your hair grows out, you'll be able to use henna (a natural hair coloring product) on it (see Chapter 9).

Rule of Thumb: If you have had a permanent wave, do **not** try to apply semipermanent colors, permanent colors or bleach to your hair at home. Consult a professional.

HOW TO DO A STRAND TEST

1. Put on rubber gloves.

2. Place a capful of the product in a small bowl (or mix it up according to the manufacturer's instructions).

3. Cut a few strands of your hair, preferably from the nape of your neck.

4. Holding securely onto the ends with one hand, dip the hair in the bowl.

5. Work the color into the hair with the fingers of the other hand.

6. Remove the hair from the bowl. (If you are using a temporary color, this is all you need to do. Now run the hair under the water to make sure that the color washes out — see page 50.)

7. Lay the hair on a small piece of plastic wrap or aluminum foil. Allow the color to develop for the time stated in the directions. Rinse the hair under the tap.

8. Dry with a paper towel. Now you have your new color.

WHAT IS THE RIGHT PRODUCT FOR YOU?

Hair coloring products are broken down into six main categories:
1. Temporary colors
2. Semipermanent colors
3. Permanent colors
4. Bleach
5. Highlighting
6. Henna

Each product has different abilities and is designed for a particular purpose.

TEMPORARY COLORS

Temporary colors are waterbased dyes and they can be a great deal of fun because unless your hair is very porous, they will wash out after only one shampoo. This means that if you have fair hair to begin with, you can be pink for an evening. The drawback to temporary colors is that they are not very strong, so you can't expect to accomplish dramatic results. Because they lie on the surface of the hair, like paint, they will only work on hair that is naturally a lighter color than the color in the bottle. They also tend to leave their mark on pillowcases, shirt collars, and so on.

Temporary colors can also help to tone down "brassy" bleached hair, or give gray hair a more silvery tone. They used to be extremely popular in hair salons. When I was working as an apprentice, nearly every customer who came into the salon with gray hair wanted a temporary color. My own feeling is that making gray hair more attractive is still their most useful role.

Today, temporary colors are much the same as they were when I started in the business. But I think this will change dramatically in the next five years. Nowadays, we have a far greater understanding of the biochemistry of hair. There's no reason why, for instance, a product couldn't be developed that would combine a hair moisturizer with a temporary color, so that you could condition your hair and try out a new color at the same time.

SEMIPERMANENT COLORS

A semipermanent color is sometimes called a rinse. It will not make your hair lighter, but it can brighten and/or darken it. A semipermanent hair color made for home-use will only last for about six to eight shampoos. **It always comes in a single bottle.** Open the box and check if you are in doubt. Otherwise you might end up putting a permanent color on your hair.

Semipermanent colors are particularly useful for coloring only the gray. Because white hair has no pigment, a woman who has, for instance, dark brown hair with some gray can blend the white hair in by using a semipermanent rinse. The white hair will color lighter than the natural dark brown (it will probably be a light brown) thus giving the hair an attractive highlight effect.

Nowadays, the quality of the colors themselves are much more natural in semipermanents than they used to be. Moreover, for professional use, manufacturers have developed a new type of semipermanent color which simultaneously conditions and colors.

PERMANENT COLORS

These are the most exciting products on the market today because they are the most versatile. Permanent colors ''tint'' your hair permanently by interacting with the natural color pigments in your hair. They will not wash out of your hair. They last until the color grows out.

What a Permanent Color Can Do

1. **Lighten:** If you want to lighten your hair at all, you will have to use a permanent color. Semipermanent and temporary colors cannot achieve this result. However, if you are lightening your hair at home, you should still stay within two levels of your natural color.

2. **Brighten:** A permanent color can add dramatic tones to your hair which would be impossible to achieve with temporary or semipermanent colors. For instance, if a woman with light brown hair (level 4) wants to become medium copper blonde (medium blonde with orange highlights — level 6) she will need to use a permanent color. A semipermanent color in the orange range would only be able to provide highlights that were in the light golden chestnut brown range (level 4).

3. **Darken:** A permanent color can darken hair and the results will look shiny and natural, never weak and dull as they would with a semipermanent or temporary color.

4. **Completely cover white hair:** A permanent color will cover white hair to the color used, although there are some rules of thumb which must be followed (see Chapter 6).

5. **Tone down hair that is too bright:** For example, hair that has been overbleached by the sun can benefit by the introduction of ash tones, as

can blonde hair that is too ''brassy''.

Adding a permanent hair color to your hair is a serious step. It should not be taken lightly. Before you commit yourself, you must consider whether your target color suits your skin tone (and your wardrobe). Moreover, since your roots will need to be retouched every four to six weeks, you must be prepared to commit the time and money to maintain your hair. Some people are just too busy. Also, if you're the kind of person who is easily bored, it might not be a good thing for you to color your hair permanently. Finally, make sure that the color you want is technically possible. If you want to be a light strawberry blonde (level 8) and your natural color is light brown (level 4) a permanent color is not for you. If you are doing it at home, you'll have to use bleach first.

BLEACHING

Bleaching is a process that strips all pigment from the hair. It will not color the hair as it lightens, so when the process is complete a light yellow results. At this point a ''toner'' (a type of semipermanent color) must be applied to the hair.

Bleach is basically ammonia, in either cream or powdered form. It is mixed with hydrogen peroxide and then applied to the hair. It has a tendency to sting when applied to the hair.

Proper bleaching is a difficult thing to do because it takes a very well-trained eye to recognize exactly where the process should stop. If it isn't stopped, the hair will eventually break off. In all my years in the business, I only saw this happen once, and it was a terrible sight to behold. The color technician in the salon where I was working was highlighting a client's hair. The hair had been pulled through a cap, bleach had been applied and the client had been placed under an infrared lamp to speed up the process. The technician became busy with something else and forgot about the customer. By the time she remembered, it was too late. She pulled off the cap and hair came with it.

If you wish to lighten your hair more than two color levels, you will either have to see your hairdresser for a "highlifting tint" or you will have to bleach your hair.

I am really not in favor of bleaching. It is very hard on the hair. It is also very time consuming and expensive to maintain, as the roots need to be redone approximately every three weeks. Before you bleach your hair you must think it through completely. Is the hair color you want really worth such an enormous amount of effort?

HIGHLIGHTS

Highlights are what the word implies – fine lights reflecting from and enhancing your natural hair color. Highlights are not bleached streaks or frosting. There are products available specifically for the home market to produce these effects.

Basically, if you're doing highlights at home they are achieved by pulling strands of hair through a highlight cap. Bleach or permanent color is applied to just these strands making them lighter or brighter than you natural color. In salons, however, highlights should be achieved by systematically separating out strands of hair, applying the color and then wrapping them with either plastic wrap or aluminum foil (see Chapter 9).

HENNA

Henna is a natural hair color that is taken from the leaves of the henna plant. It coats the hair to produce different tones of red, gold or brown. Henna is also a permanent color that will last until it grows out of the hair, although it will fade somewhat over many shampoos. There is also a neutral henna which contains no color and is used purely as a conditioner.

Rule of Thumb: It is possible to color Black and oriental hair, but caution should be exercised. The most common use of hair color is highlighting, and some dramatic effects can be achieved with blue-black and burgundy, depending on your skin tone. But see your hairdresser — don't try to color Black or oriental hair yourself.

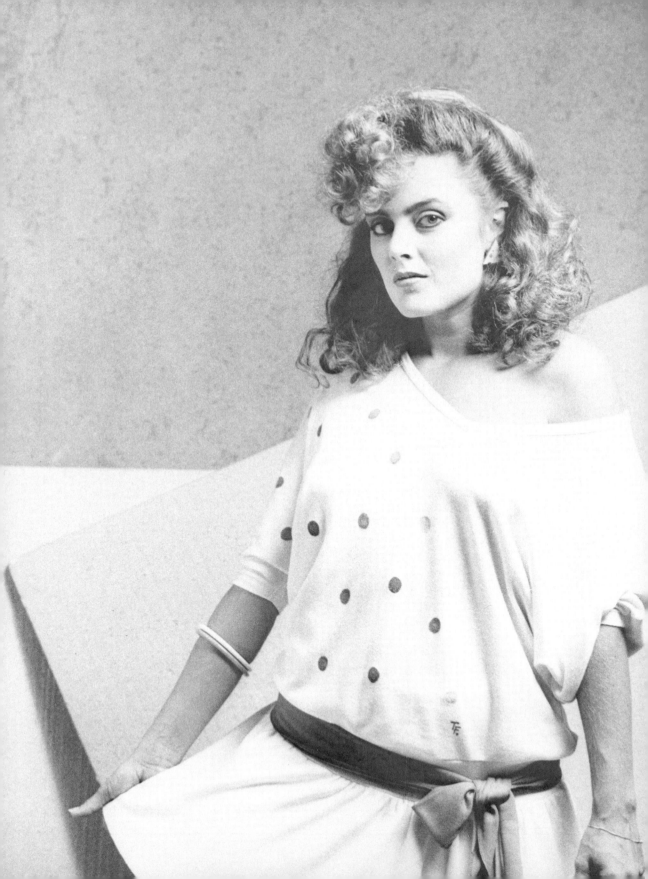

TEMPORARY AND SEMIPERMANENT COLOR

TEMPORARY AND SEMIPERMANENT COLOR

WHAT THEY ARE, WHAT THEY WILL DO AND HOW TO APPLY THEM.

Temporary and semipermanent colors have been neglected for a number of years. I suspect this is mainly because we now wash our hair much more often than we used to. In the past a woman usually went to a hair salon for a weekly wash and set. Thus, the life-span of a temporary color was a week, and a semipermanent color could be expected to last for almost two months. These days, most people wash their hair three times a week, so unless you are coloring your hair for fun, a color that will withstand a great many washings would seem preferable to one that washes out after six shampoos.

But at the same time that temporary and semipermanent colors have declined in popularity, the streets are ablaze with the most wildly artificial colors of hair — greens, pinks, purples. Largely due to the influence of punk, more and more people, even those of a generally conservative bent, are now motivated to experiment with coloring their hair. My own feeling is that this has set the stage for a renaissance in the use of temporary and semipermanent colors.

Rule of Thumb: Some people are sensitive to temporary and semipermanent colors. Therefore, all manufacturers strongly advise you to do a skin test forty-eight hours before coloring your hair (see page 41). I cannot stress the importance of this skin test too strongly. In all probability there will be no reaction. But if you are one of those rare people who is allergic to the product, you will have to relinquish the idea of coloring your hair with anything other than henna (see Chapter 9).

TEMPORARY COLOR

What Temporary Color Is
Temporary color is a water-based dye that lies on the outside of the hair shaft like paint. It will only last until you shampoo your hair again, and since it is not very potent, it's use is extremely limited.

What It Will Do
A temporary color is most useful for enhancing the appearance of gray hair, which is really a mixture of white and brown or black. Because white hair

has no pigment of its own, it is very susceptible to the influence of a temporary color. Thus a temporary color can add a silver or soft gray coating to the white hair and soften its harshness by allowing white hairs to blend slightly with the brown tones.

Temporary colors are also useful for blending in the roots when hair is very white. If, for instance, you have very white hair that has been tinted light brown or dark blonde (two tasteful choices), within two weeks you will see a white line around your hairline. You can then purchase a temporary color in a shade similar to your tint color and apply it to the white roots.

Temporary colors can be used to tone down brassy bleached hair. A temporary color in the pastel blonde tones will introduce much-needed violet to bleached hair. Still, in this case, a temporary color should only serve as an emergency measure until you can get your color corrected by a hairdresser.

These colors also offer the greatest potential for having fun with your hair color, since they should wash out, thus, you can color your hair black and become a vampire for Halloween, or go green for St. Patrick's day.

Warning: If you're using a temporary color for fun, you must make certain that you don't have porous hair (hair that has the ability to absorb liquid at a particularly fast rate). Therefore, as with any other kind of color, you should do a strand test before using a temporary color if you want it to wash out. Allow the color to process on your test strand for the required amount of time, then run it under water. If it rinses out of the strand completely, then you can have fun hair.

Disadvantages: I've known lots of women whose whole personality has been brightened up by the use of a temporary color. Still, they do have disadvantages. Because they coat the surface of the hair, they do not allow light to pass through, which means they tend to have a hard and unnatural look. This is particularly true if you are using them to achieve dramatic results — for instance, coloring your light brown hair black for Halloween.

Moreover, because a temporary color lies on the outside of the hair shaft, it also tends to come off very easily. You will see traces of the color on your pillow or hair brush. And if, by chance, your hair gets wet in the rain, the color will rinse out. This could be particularly troublesome if you were wearing a white blouse. If this does happen, rinse the fabric in cold water as soon as possible, or have it dry cleaned immediately. Because temporary colors are very gentle, I have never heard of a case where they permanently stained a fabric.

Rule of Thumb: Temporary colors will only work on hair that is naturally lighter than the color in the bottle.

HOW TO APPLY TEMPORARY COLOR

What You Need

shampoo

towel

surgical gloves

temporary color in applicator bottle

wide-tooth comb

To Prepare

1. At least 48 hours before coloring your hair, do a sensitivity test and a strand test to make certain that the color will wash out of your hair (see pages 41 and 42).

2. Just before coloring, shampoo and towel dry your hair. Do not use a conditioner (cream rinse) as it could form a barrier to the color. Most temporary colors include a conditioner of their own.

3. Put on your surgical gloves.

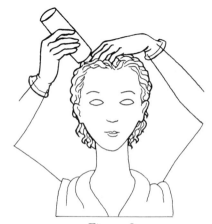

Figure 3

To Color

1. Shake the applicator bottle and release the nozzle in the cap. Invert the bottle and touch the nozzle to the hair near your scalp.

2. Gently press the sides of the bottle, releasing the rinse in gentle spurts. With your other hand, simultaneously massage the rinse into the hair nearest the scalp (Figure 3).

3. Continue applying the rinse in frequent spurts all over your scalp, massaging it in as you go. This should take about two minutes.

4. Comb the rinse through your hair (Figure 4).

To Finish

1. Dry and style your hair. You do not rinse the temporary color out of your hair.

Rule of Thumb: If you are using a temporary color on hair that has been bleached, comb the color through the hair but leave out the ends. The blonde hair on the end will be more porous than on the rest of the hair shaft, causing it to absorb more of the color and resulting in a different shade.

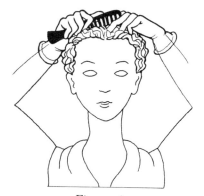

Figure 4

SEMIPERMANENT COLOR

Semipermanent colors first became popular in the Sixties when women usually visited their hairdressers for a weekly wash and set. So in those days, a semipermanent rinse that lasted for six shampoos remained in the hair for about six weeks. Nowadays, hair is likely to get washed three times a week, so, like temporary colors, semipermanent rinses have declined in popularity.

Nevertheless, there are some semipermanent rinses (available only for professional use) which will remain in the hair for six to eight weeks, even if it is washed almost every other day. Moreover, these new semipermanents can accomplish some quite breathtaking results. The colors contain remarkable conditioners and the tint itself is not flat and heavy. These new semipermanents give the hair what we call *luminosity*, because they allow light to pass through the hair. These salon semipermanents soften the outside of the hair (the cuticle) and are absorbed into these outside layers, though they do not penetrate the whole shaft as permanent colors do. Herein lies the secret of their high degree of brilliance which even many permanent colors can't match.

Semipermanent colors used to be the conventional way of introducing a client to color. But today they are often neglected in salons because many hairdressers prefer to use highlights or henna.

I'm very fond of semipermanent colors and I use them a lot in the salon. They are a great introduction to color since they only take three minutes to apply and twenty minutes to develop. This means that a client can see results in less than half an hour. A good semipermanent color has the potential to transform a nonbeliever into a color disciple for life.

Semipermanent colors are improving at such a rapid rate that I'm convinced that their popularity will increase. The manufacturers who provide products to the salons are beginning to emphasize their new semipermanent colors. Eventually this influence will filter through to the general public. That graying baby boom is waiting to be introduced to hair color, and semipermanent color is probably the best place to start.

What Semipermanent Color Is

Like temporary colors, semipermanent colors lie on the outside of the hair. But they seep through several layers of the cuticle, which is the source of their staying power for more than one shampoo. Basically, the products themselves are a mixture of water, color, a mild soap to induce lather and some form of conditioner.

Rule of Thumb: A semipermanent color is always a single-bottle product. If in doubt, open the box and check. I can't tell you the number of times that clients have arrived at the salon convinced that they've only used a "rinse" which will wash out, when in fact they have used a permanent color kit, which includes a second bottle containing hydrogen peroxide. Semipermanent colors in the form of foam have recently been introduced to the home market. These are an improvement over the existing products as they are easier to apply and the colors don't drip.

What Semipermanent Color Will Do

A semipermanent color made for home use will last for six to eight shampoos. It will not lighten your hair but it will make it darker or brighter. If you have gray hair, it will color to about 70 percent of the color described on the box. If you don't have gray hair, it will color to the color described, provided that your hair is *lighter* than your color choice. Therefore, color choice is simple. As long as the color is as dark as, or no more than two levels darker than your natural color (see page 26), you can use any color you wish.

Rule of Thumb: You shouldn't try to go more than two levels darker with a semipermanent color. This is asking it to do too much and the results can look hard and unnatural. If you want to darken your hair by more than two levels, I advise that you use a permanent color, but check with your hairdresser.

Unfortunately, the use of semipermanent colors to improve gray hair is now a neglected area. The newer products can blend gray hair with a natural hair color effectively and naturally. For instance, a soft, smoky ash color will enhance gray hair, making it look very pretty.

HOW TO APPLY
SEMIPERMANENT COLOR

What You Need

semipermanent color kit (This will contain
bottle of color, shampoo, conditioner, gloves
and plastic cap.)

petroleum jelly

thin strips of cotton batting, 12 inches long

towel

To Prepare

1. At least 48 hours before coloring your hair, do a
sensitivity test and a strand test (see pages 41 and
42).

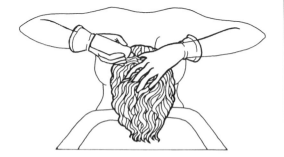

Figure 5

2. Just before coloring, wet your hair and towel it
dry. Although the instruction sheet that comes
with your semipermanent color may tell you to
apply the color to dry hair, I have found that the
performance improves if it is applied to wet hair. If
you have not washed your hair in more than three
days, I recommend that you give it a light shampoo
first as well. Otherwise natural oils and per-
spiration might form a barrier between your hair
and the color, and you may not get the best results.

3. Put on your gloves.

4. Smear a half-inch band of petroleum jelly
around your hairline and ears. This will protect
your skin from becoming the same color as your
hair.

To Color

1. Leaning over a bath or basin, pour a small
amount of semipermanent color onto your hair.

2. With your free hand, massage the color through your hair. Work in circular movements, pouring small amounts of color and massaging the color simultaneously (Figure 5).

3. When you think you have colored all the hair, put the bottle down and, with both hands, massage the color throughout your hair to ensure that you haven't missed any spots.

4. Rinse the color off your gloves. Place the cotton batting on top of the petroleum jelly all around your hairline. Tuck the loose ends under.

5. Place the plastic cap over your head. To make sure it fits snugly, take an open end at the edge of the cap and gently twist it tight. Slip the edge back under the cap. It will not loosen (Figure 6).

6. Let the color develop according to the package instructions.

7. Remove the plastic cap and cotton batting. Have the shampoo and conditioner ready for use (if you need to cut the top off a plastic packet, do so before you rinse off the color).

8. Add water to your hair and lather it up, or apply the shampoo/conditioner provided (depending on the manufacturer's instructions). Some products provide shampoo and conditioner. In others, the color itself becomes a shampoo once you add water to it. In some kits the conditioner should remain on the hair, whereas other advise that you wash it off. So it is important to read the instructions that come with your kit very carefully (Figure 7).

To Finish

1. Dry and style your hair.

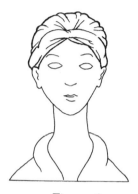

Figure 6

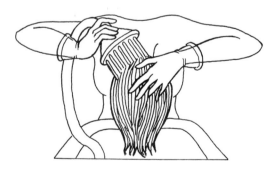

Figure 7

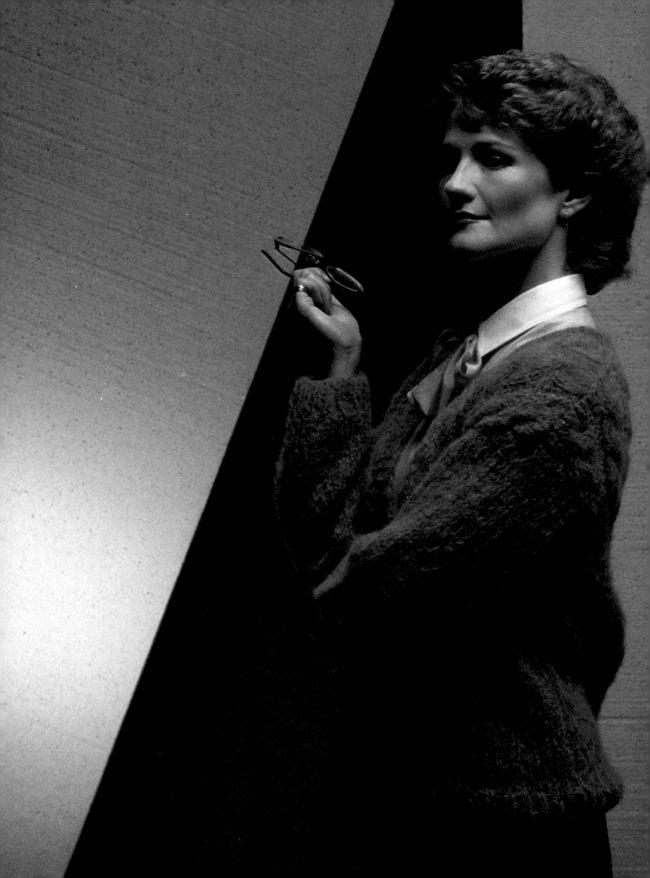

PERMANENT COLOR

PERMANENT COLOR

WHAT IT IS AND WHAT IT WILL DO; WHEN NOT TO USE A PERMANENT COLOR; HOW TO LIGHTEN YOUR HAIR USING PERMANENT COLOR; TINTING REGROWTH; TIPS ON GOING RED, GOING BROWN AND COLORING GRAY AND WHITE HAIR. HOW TO APPLY PERMANENT COLOR.

In a sense, we have come full circle in the kind of permanent colors we use today. In the 1950's, permanent colors were very thick cream, which had to be mixed with hydrogen peroxide. Not only was this a very hard job — almost like mixing a thick paste without water — but because of the heaviness of the cream and the harshness of the dyes, the hair colors were very strong and they didn't have much shine.

In the early 1960's all this changed with the development of gel — or oil-based colors. Now the color could be added to an equal amount of hydrogen peroxide and within ten seconds we had a manageable gel. Perhaps even more important, because the color itself was more translucent, permanent color had the ability to create shiny hair.

With the advent of these gels, came another way of applying color. Instead of using a brush, hairdressers began to use a plastic applicator bottle with a long nozzle and fine hole at the end. This meant that the color could be squeezed onto the hair with one hand while the thumb of the other hand gently pushed the color into the hair. This method is still used in many salons throughout North America today (in Europe and Australia colors are still usually applied with a brush). It is also the method recommended for people who color their hair at home.

However, even the gels could be improved upon, with the result that over the past fifteen years a superior cream-based color has been developed. Not only does it have the capacity to color and to condition the hair better than gels, but the cream itself softens the hair and is chemically biodegradable, which means that it can be absorbed by the hair. In the last two years these new cream-based products have become available for the home market.

What Permanent Color Is

A permanent color (tint) is a cream- or gel-based dye which is mixed with hydrogen peroxide. Once it is applied to the hair and allowed to process for the proper amount of time, it is permanent. The only way to remove the color from the hair is to grow it or cut it out of the hair.

A permanent color is easily distinguished from a temporary or semipermanent hair color because each kit always contains two bottles. One bottle contains hydrogen peroxide; the other contains the "color" tint plus ammonia. The contents of these two bottles must be mixed together before the product will work.

When these products are mixed together, a process known as oxidation occurs. As the mixture is applied to hair, each strand expands so that the color moves inside the hair, staining natural color granules with the artificial pigments. A tint, therefore, is not like a can of paint that will color any surface with the color you buy. A tint needs to work with the natural tones of your hair because it combines with them to produce another color. This is why it is so crucial to understand the nature of color and to know exactly what your natural color is before you try to change the color of your hair.

What Permanent Color Will Do

A permanent color can do four basic things:

1. **Lighten**. Unlike a temporary or semi-permanent color, permanent color can lighten hair. At the same time as it lightens, it can add color to the hair, as opposed to a bleach which will only strip color from hair (see Chapter 7). If you want to lighten your hair at home, the permanent hair color products available will allow you to accurately predict the end result provided that your target color is within two levels lighter on the color chart (see page 26).

2. **Darken**. No matter what color you are to begin with, a permanent color can technically darken your hair to any color. However, if you are coloring hair at home you should generally not try to darken your hair by more than two levels. Skin tone, lifestyle, etc., should also be considered (see Chapter 3).

3. **Brighten**. A permanent color can brighten your hair by adding warm tones (red, gold, orange) whether they be on a lighter level, the same level or a darker level.

4. **Completely cover gray**. A permanent color will completely change white hair to the color used. But because white hair has no pigment of its own, certain rules of thumb must be considered in the selection of color.

5. **Tone down hair that is too bright**. A permanent color can tone down hair. If, for instance, your hair has become too bright from being out in the sun, or too brassy, the addition of ash tones will correct the problem.

WHEN NOT TO USE A PERMANENT COLOR

1. If you have done the sensitivity test and had an allergic reaction.

2. If you have cuts or abrasions on your scalp.

3. Over permanent waves at home. (Even in the salon we only use permanent color over a permanent wave if the hair is of good quality and in good condition.)

4. Over hennaed hair. Henna coats the hair and, therefore, forms a barrier that is very difficult to break down. Moreover, the red that lies on the surface has also been absorbed by the hair as the henna processed. Applying permanent color will result in the oxidation of an extra red pigment. This will produce an undesirable color. Wait until the henna has grown out before applying a permanent color.

5. If you have been taking prescription drugs over a long period of time (more than sixty days) or are on chemotherapy, you might have a problem. There's a possibility that the drug has altered the chemical balance of your hair, affecting your ability to predict your target color accurately. So do a strand test, using hair from above the ear and the nape of your neck. If the chemical balance of your hair has been affected, it either won't color at all, or will go an entirely different color from the one you intended.

6. Over previously tinted hair. If your hair already has permanent, semipermanent or temporary color on it, do not try to tint your hair at home. Wait until the previous color has grown out or been washed out, or see your hairdresser.

Rule of Thumb: If your hair is over six inches long, always buy a second hair color kit. You may need it to cover your head fully. If not, save it. You can use it for the next application.

HOW TO LIGHTEN YOUR HAIR USING PERMANENT COLOR

The first thing to remember about lightening your hair at home is that if the color is applied all at once, your roots will become much lighter than the ends of your hair. This is because your scalp generates heat which causes the color to process at a more rapid rate. This is why you should use a special technique when applying color to hair that is to be lightened. The method I've outlined is time consuming, but it's essential if you want a nice even color all over your head. Over the years, I've had many customers who have lightened their hair at home by throwing the color on all at once. The color at the roots is the one they want to achieve, perhaps a light ash blonde, but the middle part of the hair is a rather unattractive yellow and the ends are gold.

If it seems like too much effort to apply the color in stages, then you can either go to your hairdresser who will do it for you, or choose a color that's on the same level as your natural color and forget about going lighter.

Rule of Thumb: The longer your hair is, the more important it is to apply the color in stages. If your hair is eight inches long there's a dramatic difference in the processing time between the ends and the roots. The results will be very unattractive. But if your hair is only two inches long, obviously you're not going to experience a problem.

If you feel that it is too difficult for you to follow the instructions for applying permanent color by yourself, why not have a hair coloring party? You're bound to produce better results with the help of a friend.

What You Need

hair color kit (This will contain tint, peroxide, gloves, shampoo and conditioner. One of the bottles also acts as the applicator bottle.)

towels

petroleum jelly

paper tissues

To Prepare

1. At least 48 hours before coloring your hair, do a sensitivity test and a strand test (see pages 41 and 42).

2. In the bathroom or kitchen, lay out everything you will need.

3. Put on your gloves.

4. Smear petroleum jelly around your hairline, neck and ears.

5. Cut off the tip of the nozzle on the applicator bottle. Pour the contents of the other bottle into the applicator bottle. Place your finger over the nozzle, invert the bottle and shake the solutions together for a few seconds. They will form a creamy gel.

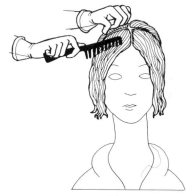

Figure 8

To Color

1. Divide your hair into four quarters by parting your hair down the middle from forehead to neck and from ear to ear (Figure 8).

2. Apply the color on the right hand back section first. Make 1/4-inch diagonal partings, beginning at the nape of the neck, and apply the color on the middle lengths and ends of the hair, leaving about 1-1/2 inches of hair nearest the scalp free of color (Figure 9).

3. Continue coloring each parting, all the way up to the crown.

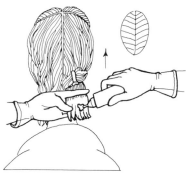

Figure 9

4. Repeat on the left side of the back section.

5. Starting at the temple, make 1/4-inch partings diagonally across the right hand front section and apply color to the middle lengths and ends. Do not color the 1-1/2 inches of hair nearest the scalp. Continue until you reach the crown (Figure 10).

6. Repeat the procedures on the right hand side of the front section.

7. Allow the color to develop for about 15 minutes.

8. Now apply the remaining color to the 1-1/2 inches of hair next to the scalp. Start at the nape of the neck again and take the same partings as before.

9. When all your hair is colored, gently scrunch all the hair together and add the color remaining in the bottle. Make sure the color is evenly distributed (Figure 11).

10. Allow the color to develop another 15 minutes.

11. Check a few strands of hair by wiping them clean with a paper tissue to see if they are the same color from the scalp through to the ends. If they aren't, leave the color on for another 10 minutes and then check again.

12. When the hair is an even color, add water to the color and lather. Rinse until the water runs clear.

To Finish

1. Shampoo your hair with the product provided, or use a high-quality protein shampoo and moisturizer (see Chapter 9).

2. Towel dry your hair.

3. Clean up and throw away both bottles. If any color remains, it will not be reusable. If the towel or basin are stained, simply wash them with soap and water.

4. Dry and style your hair.

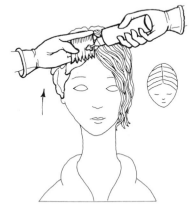

Figure 10

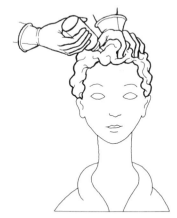

Figure 11

TINTING YOUR REGROWTH

About three or four weeks after you have tinted your hair you will see your natural color growing through. This regrowth is often incorrectly referred to as "roots" (the roots of your hair are inside your head).

Tinting your regrowth is a more involved process than you might think. In the instructions that come with your hair color, you will find that the procedure for every application is the same, whether it is the first time you are coloring your hair or the 101st. However, I believe that there is bound to be a certain amount of deterioration in the porosity of your hair if you're applying color to it every four to six weeks. You may not notice this immediately, but you will definitely be aware of a difference after six months.

The gradual deterioration of hair that is constantly colored is, in part, the cause of the loss in shine which creates what people describe as the "dyed" look. Tinted hair should not look dry and unnatural. Indeed, with the quality of products that are available today, it should have a glowing, healthy and natural-looking shine. Using my method for tinting regrowth, your hair should always be in the best possible condition and your color should always look completely natural.

To Prepare

1. Purchase the same color you used for the previous application.

2. Do a sensitivity test (see page 41).

3. Assemble the same materials as the last time (see page 61).

4. Put on your gloves.

5. Smear petroleum jelly around your hairline, the back of the neck and ears.

6. Snip the tip off the nozzle on the applicator bottle and mix the colors as you did with your previous tint application.

To Color

1. Separate your hair into four quarters by taking a parting down the middle of your hair from the forehead to the base of the neck. Then part from ear to ear.

2. Start applying your color at the nape of the neck on the right hand quarter. Taking 1/4-inch partings, **apply the color to your regrowth only.**

3. Continue with 1/4-inch partings, applying color to the regrowth only on all of the right back section.

4. Proceed as above for the other three sections of your head, working towards the crown on the front section.

5. If the total development time stated on the package of color is 20 minutes, allow 15 minutes to pass. Then work the remainder of color in the bottle through to the ends of your hair. This should take about 1 minute. Leave your hair for another 4 minutes. If your color needs 30 minutes to develop, allow 25 minutes before working the color through to the ends of the hair. Again, allow it to develop for a final 4 minutes.

To Finish

1. Shampoo with the shampoo and conditioner provided. If they are not provided, use a high-quality protein shampoo and protein moisturizer (see Chapter 9).

GOING RED

Aside from blonde, the second favorite hair color is a tone of red, whether a red-gold, orange-red or a true deep red. The permanent color products on the market today in the red tones will help you achieve these results, as long as you follow the guidelines outlined here and in Chapter 3. With women under thirty, I sometimes break my own rules, especially with reds. For instance, if someone has very light blonde hair and delicate skin tones, she could look fantastic as a rich medium copper blonde, although it's a very dramatic change. The problems with coloring hair red result more often from making hair lighter and redder. However, if you want to use red to make this kind of radical change, consult with your hairdresser. The red pigments in the tint could combine with the red, orange, gold and yellow pigments in your natural hair color to produce an undesireable result.

Rule of Thumb: Keep within one level either lighter or darker than your natural color if you are using reds. The intensity of the color you choose depends upon considerations such as lifestyle and skin tones.

GOING BROWN

Most women with neutral brown hair usually only want a subtle change in their natural hair color. They don't want their hair to look mousy, but at the same time, they don't want to have red, orange or gold in their hair. Nor do they want to be blondes. All they want is to be a nicer brown than they are.

Hairdressers love to justify the fact that they are very creative people. Often they seem offended when confronted with a client who asks for something which is just a very simple modification to the color of their hair. Their response is likely to be "Why did you come to *me* if you only wanted to do *that?*"

And yet, achieving a subtle change which is only noticeable to the client is just as creative and can, in fact, bc more difficult than changing her into a dramatic redhead or a beautiful blonde. Brown, too, can be beautiful.

My rule of thumb for these clients is to keep their new color as close to their natural color as possible. Therefore, we usually go either only one level lighter or darker than their natural color.

If you want your brown hair to remain almost the same color as your natural color, I would recommend that you either use an identical color to your natural color which will, in fact, make your hair appear slightly darker and certainly deeper in tone, *or* use a color just one level lighter than your natural color, which will change your mousy brown hair into a softer brown. If you decide that you want a slightly more noticeable change, then you can add gold tones, either at the same level or one level up from the color you previously used.

The advantage to coloring your hair brown is that you won't notice much regrowth. After about ten weeks the hair nearest the scalp will only appear duller than the rest of your hair. This is the time to recolor (see pages 63 to 64).

COLORING GRAY OR WHITE HAIR

You'll likely remember that gray hair is, in fact, an optical illusion created when white hairs mix with brown or black.

This means that if you're coloring your gray hair at home, you should stay within the neutral tones. It's the only time we can compare using a permanent hair color to a coat of paint. If you apply light brown to white hair, light brown will result.

The difficulty in coloring white hair shows up when we use a color that has a strong pigment i.e. red, gold or orange. Because the white hair has no pigment of its own, it will take on the character of the dominant pigment being used and very undesirable colors can result.

Say, for instance, you are a medium copper blonde with 50 percent white. Now, mixed with the white, your hair appears to be a very light copper blonde. While realizing that you can't turn the clock back twenty years and become the color you used to be, you would like to achieve a color similar to your original color. To achieve this, you might, quite logically, apply a light copper blonde tint to your hair. This would be a mistake. The dominant orange pigment in the color would be much more than you need, with the result that your hair would resemble a bright pink-orange sunset — definitely not what you had in mind.

To achieve the result you want, you will need to weaken the orange. The only way to do this is to purchase a second color from the neutral category at the same level (light blonde). Mix them together in equal proportions. This will reduce the copper by half.

Rule of Thumb: If your natural hair color has a predominant tone, and you want to add this tone to your gray hair, always mix the color with equal proportions of the neutral color of the same level as your target color.

HOW TO APPLY PERMANENT COLOR ON RED, BROWN OR GRAY HAIR, OR BLONDE HAIR THAT IS NOT BEING LIGHTENED

What you Need

hair color kit (This will contain tint, peroxide, gloves, shampoo and conditoner. One of the bottles also serves as an applicator bottle.)

towels

petroleum jelly

paper tissues

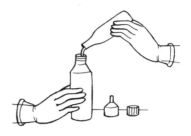

Figure 12

To Prepare

1. At least 48 hours before you intend to apply permanent color to your hair, do a sensitivity test and a strand test (see pages 41 and 42).

2. In the bathroom or the kitchen, lay out everything you need in front of you.

3. Put on your gloves.

4. Smear petroleum jelly around your hairline, neck and ears.

5. Snip the tip of the nozzle on the applicator bottle with a pair of scissors. Pour the contents of the other bottle into the applicator bottle (Figure 12). Place a finger tip over the hole of the nozzle, invert the bottle and shake the solutions together for a few seconds. They will form a creamy gel.

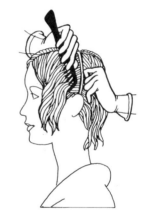

Figure 13

To Color

1. Divide your hair into four quarters by parting your hair down the middle from forehead to neck and from ear to ear (Figure 13).

2. Start applying the color on the left hand quarter of the back sections first. Make 1/4-inch diagonal partings, beginning at the nape of the neck, and apply the color to the hair (Figure 14).

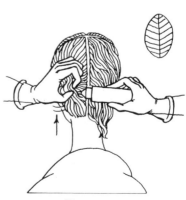

Figure 14

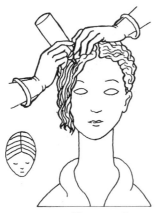

Figure 15

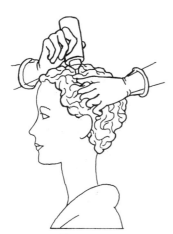

Figure 16

3. Continue taking 1/4-inch partings all the way up to the crown.

4. Repeat on the right side of the back section.

5. Starting at the temple, take 1/4-inch partings diagonally across the right hand front section and apply color to the hair. Continue until you reach the crown.

6. Repeat the procedure on the left hand side of the front section (Figure 15).

7. When all the hair is colored, gently scrunch all the hair together and add the color remaining in the bottle. Make sure the color is evenly distributed (Figure 16).

8. Allow the color to develop for the required amount of time. To check the color, wipe a few strands of hair clean with a paper tissue.

9. Add water to the color and lather. Rinse until the water runs clear.

To Finish
1. Shampoo with the product provided. If none is provided, use a high-quality protein shampoo and moisturizer (see Chapter 9).
2. Towel dry your hair.
3. Clean up and throw away both bottles. If any color remains, it will not be reusable. If the towel or basin are stained, simply wash them with soap and water.
4. Dry and style your hair.

TINTING YOUR REGROWTH

Depending on how dramatically you have altered your natural color, from four to ten weeks after you have tinted your hair, you will see your natural color growing through. This "regrowth" will have to be tinted to match the rest of your head. To do this, follow the instructions on pages 63 to 64.

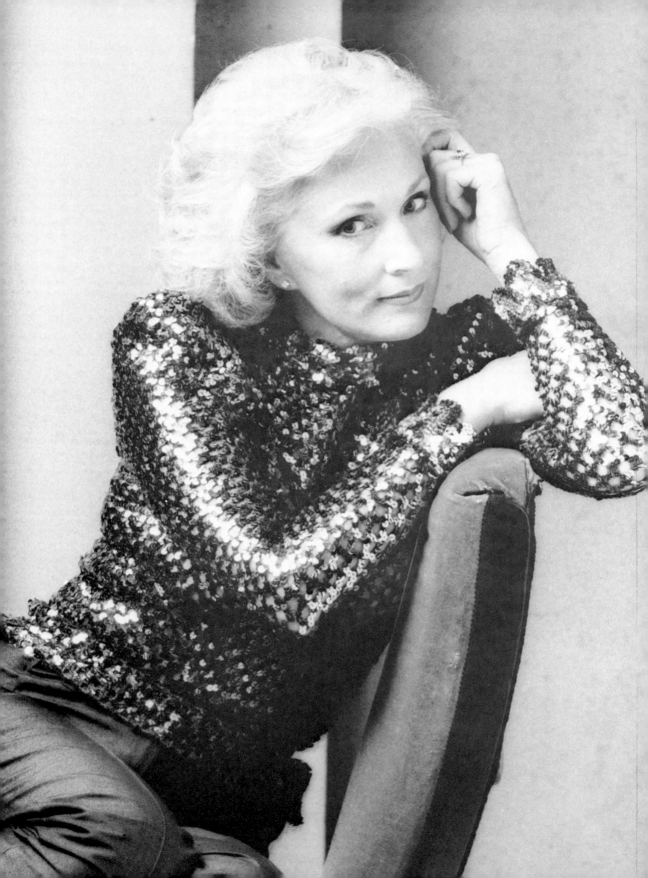

BLEACH

BLEACH

WHAT IT IS AND WHAT IT WILL DO; THINGS TO CONSIDER BEFORE APPLYING BLEACH; WHEN NOT TO BLEACH. HOW TO APPLY BLEACH AND TONER.

Bleaching has fallen out of fashion in recent years, but I firmly believe that it's due for a renaissance of sorts. The practice of bleaching the entire head may not return, but I do think that our greater knowledge of color as it relates to light will enable us to use bleach rather as an artist uses white to focus the eye or to reduce a color. My own feeling is that we'll begin to use bleach on different sections of the head, combining it with permanent color to create graduating tones of blonde throughout the hair.

I have a client who not long ago was auditioning for a television show. Although her hair was a natural light brown (level 4) the producers demanded that she become a very light golden blonde (level 8). This was the hair color of the woman who had previously held the position and they wanted to maintain the tradition. Against my better judgement, I bleached her hair, and six hours later she was a pastel golden blonde. Her skin tones, I might add, were pink and the two colors clashed, making her hair look more yellow than it actually was. But the producers loved it and my client went off to meet her boyfriend and some of his business associates for dinner.

This woman is usually very calm and level headed. But the next morning I got a call from her and she was practically hysterical.

"I can't believe that the color of my hair could make such a difference to the way people treat me," she moaned. "I've known these people for years, and they've always respected and admired the way I looked and dressed. Suddenly they were making cheap remarks and giving me looks that made me feel like a hooker."

She was devastated and unable to face anyone, let alone a television camera, until I had changed her hair back to a more acceptable color. Fortunately I was able to achieve a shade of blonde that satisfied everyone. However, I tell you the story to make one simple but very crucial point: it can be a traumatic experience to become a blonde when you're naturally a brunette.

I don't want you to underestimate the difference this will make in your life. Not only is going from light brown to light blonde a dramatic change, but you must also prepare yourself for the fact that it does not look natural. Virtually all the pigments in your hair have been stripped away and it takes on a pastel appearance. It can look stunningly beautiful, but it is definitely different.

This point is very important because such a dramatic change will affect the way other people will look at you and feel about you. Such a radical change in your appearance may be construed as an aggressive act, and people may react in a hostile way. So warn your husband, boyfriend, friends, family or whomever you care about, first. It's a good idea to talk it over with them before you do actually bleach your hair — they may have very strong feelings that you should stay just the way you are.

What Bleaching Is

Bleaching is a completely different process from the ones we have discussed. Unlike the results achieved with temporary, semipermanent or permanent colors, bleaching does not add color to the hair. In fact, a bleach will remove all natural pigments from the hair. It does not create any color other than yellow.

A bleach can lighten any natural color — even black — to a very pale yellow. But this is extremely inadvisable. Moreover, this pale yellow is, in itself, an undesirable color. So after the hair is bleached, we must add an acceptable shade of blonde with a *toner*.

A toner is a semipermanent or permanent color that comes in a variety of pastel blonde tones. I prefer toners that don't need peroxide (there are two kinds), not only because they will not sting an already sensitive scalp, but also because they can be used to freshen up the color between bleaches without altering the color of the regrowth. When a peroxide toner is used between bleaches, it will lift the red pigments out of the regrowth, leaving a red rim around the hair.

What It Will Do

Bleaching is only done when a dramatic change is required, that is to say, if you want to become *very* blonde and your target color is more than two levels lighter than your natural color according to the chart on page 26. However, if you want to lighten your hair by more than two levels, rather than bleaching it at home, I strongly advise that you see your hairdresser who may be able to achieve the level of blondeness you want by using a highlifting tint. It is a much better way of going blonde because it is not as hard on your hair.

THINGS TO CONSIDER BEFORE BLEACHING

1. **The condition of your hair**. The hair should be in excellent condition before you start because bleaching will dry out the hair.

2. **The texture of your hair.** I would not advise someone with fine hair or with thick, coarse hair to bleach. Normally fragile hair will become even more fragile.

3. **The elasticity of the hair.** Test the elasticity of your hair by pulling out a strand and then stretching it between your fingers. If it breaks or doesn't stretch to more than half its length again and spring back to its correct length, your hair is not strong enough. If your hair is bleached, it will break just with regular brushing or combing.

4. **The maintenance involved**. Because of the contrast between your natural hair color and the shade of blonde you have chosen, regrowth is extremely noticeable on bleached hair (within five days). To maintain your color properly, therefore, you will need to bleach the regrowth every three weeks. Bleaching and toning hair every three weeks will take about 1-1/2 to 2 hours. Because of the time, amount of product used and, most importantly, the knowledge which goes into bleaching your hair, the cost will be considerable if it's done at a salon. In addition, you will have to take special care of your hair at home by using only high-quality hair products.

Rule of Thumb: The condition of your hair prior to bleaching has to be excellent. Fine hair darker than dark blonde will easily break before achieving the desired level of lightness so it shouldn't be bleached.

WHEN NOT TO BLEACH

1. Do not bleach hair that has been chemically altered because it has been permed, previously tinted or has henna on it. (The artificial pigments will have to be removed before the real stripping of the natural pigments can begin and artificial pigments are more difficult to remove.)

2. Do not bleach if you have cuts or abrasions on your scalp. Bleaching can be very painful to your scalp.

Rule of Thumb: To bleach virgin hair (hair that has not been previously altered by a permanent wave, permanent tint or henna), you must set aside a whole day. It takes at least six hours to apply and process bleach through the necessary stages. Another hour is required for the toner.

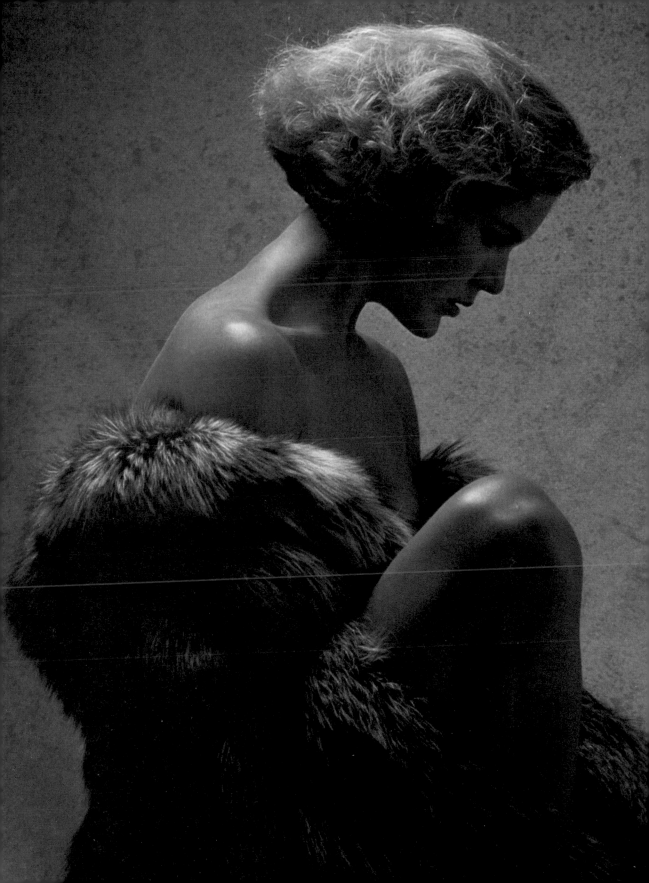

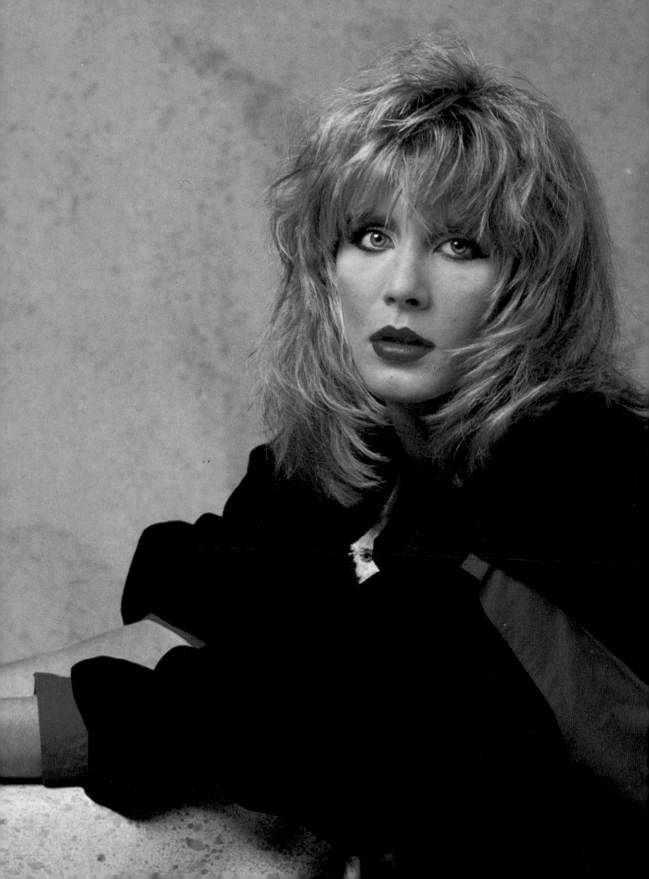

HOW TO APPLY BLEACH AND TONER

What You Need

hair bleach, at least 8 ounces (The kit will contain liquid and two sachets containing a powdered bleaching agent. Mixing these will create a creamy bleach which is what you need. Make sure that you do not use a powdered bleach, which is more difficult to apply and much harsher on the hair.)

hydrogen peroxide, 16 ounces (20 volume)

2 pairs plastic gloves (in case one rips)

plastic clips

petroleum jelly

applicator bottle

towels

shampoo and conditioner

paper tissues

cotton batting (Buy a roll of cotton and make yourself 3 wide strips approximately 3 inches wide and 12 inches long; and 70 narrow strips approximately 1/4 inch wide and 5 inches long.)

toner kit (This will include toner, crystals, gloves and conditioner. One of the bottles will act as an applicator.)

To Prepare

1. At least 48 hours before bleaching your hair, do a sensitivity test using the toner (see page 41). There is no dye in the bleach so it is not necessary to do a sensitivity test with this product. You must also do two separate strand tests, one for just the bleach and one for the bleach and the toner (see page 42). Keep these test strands. The toner will determine what level you will bleach you hair to – yellow, pale yellow or very pale yellow. The proper level will be marked on the box.

2. In the bathroom or kitchen, lay out everything you will need (for both bleaching and toning) in front of you.

3. Put on your gloves.

4. Smear petroleum jelly around your hairline, neck and ears.

5. To prepare bleach, pour 4 ounces of peroxide into the bleach applicator bottle.

6. Snip a corner of each sachet and tip the contents into the applicator bottle (Figure 17).

7. Hold the tip of the nozzle firmly and gently shake the peroxide and powders together.

8. Unscrew the nozzle and pour 2 ounces of the blue liquid (oil bleach) into the applicator bottle (Figure 17). Place your finger over the tip of the nozzle, invert the bottle and shake the mixture vigorously until it becomes a creamy gel. Remove your finger slowly, otherwise the bleach may spurt out.

9. Prepare the toner by pouring the crystals into the toner applicator bottle (Figure 18). Shake the bottle to mix.

Figure 17

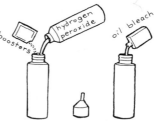

Figure 18

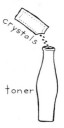

To Bleach

1. Divide the hair into four equal sections by making a part from the crown to the nape, and another from ear to ear (Figure 19).

2. Start applying the bleach on the left hand quarter of the back sections by making 1/4-inch partings, beginning at the nape of the neck. Apply the bleach on the middle lengths and ends of the hair, leaving about 1-1/2 inches of hair nearest the scalp free of bleach (Figure 20).

3. Place a narrow strip of cotton between each parting after applying the bleach. This will help to lift each parting up and away from the scalp. It will also protect the unbleached hair from becoming bleached (Figure 21).

4. Continue bleaching 1/4-inch partings until you reach the crown.

5. Repeat on the right side of the back section.

6. Take a wide strip of cotton and place it underneath the bleached hair at the back of the neck. This will give your skin greater protection from the bleach.

7. Now, starting at the temple, take 1/4-inch partings diagonally across the right hand front section and apply bleach to the middle lengths and ends (Figure 22). Once again, place narrow strips of cotton between each part.

8. Continue bleaching 1/4-inch partings until you reach the crown.

9. Place a thick strip of cotton under the first parting at the temple to protect your face from the bleach (Figure 23).

10. Repeat the procedure on the left hand side of

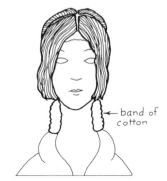

band of cotton

Figure 19

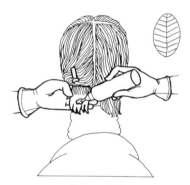

Figure 20

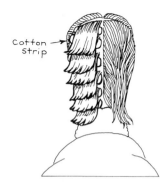

Cotton strip

Figure 21

the front section.

11. Allow the bleach to stay on your hair until it has reached a gold color (up to two hours). This color will represent about half the degree of lightness you wish to achieve. The next stage will be to apply the bleach to the remainder of your virgin hair, but first you should remove the bleach already on your hair. I have found it is best to apply a fresh bleach to the middle lengths and ends so that the hair will lighten evenly from now on, from scalp to ends. (Remember, the bleach on your ends has been there for one to two hours already. If you only applied fresh bleach to the hair nearest your scalp now, it will have two hours of power plus heat from your head to help it process. The ends won't be able to catch up with it, and they won't be light enough.)

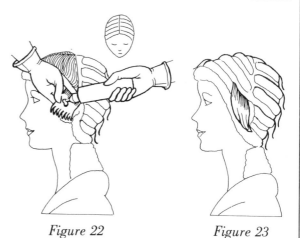

Figure 22   Figure 23

12. Remove all the cotton strips and rinse the old bleach thoroughly off the hair with water (Figure 24).

13. Towel dry the hair.

14. Mix fresh bleach as previously described.

15. Reapply the petroleum jelly.

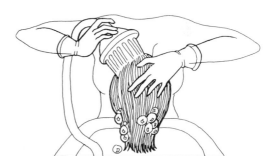

Figure 24

16. Put gloves on again.

17. Section the hair into 4 quarters as before.

18. Begin applying the bleach, starting at the nape and taking the same 1/4-inch partings. Holding the applicator bottle in your hand, apply the bleach to the virgin hair nearest the scalp (Figure 25). With the edge of the thumb of your other hand, evenly distribute the bleach **up to the previously bleached hair.**

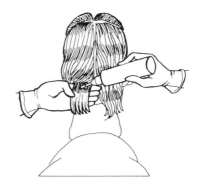

Figure 25

19. Continue the application process working toward the crown.

20. Repeat the procedure on the other side of the back section.

21. Now, starting at the temple, take 1/4-inch partings diagonally across the left hand front section and apply the bleach to the virgin hair in the same manner as the back sections.

22. Continue taking 1/4-inch partings until you reach the crown.

23. Repeat the procedure on the right hand front section (Figure 26).

24. Rinse the bleach off your gloves (keep them on your hands) and dry them.

25. Determine how much bleach you used for the previous application to the middle lengths and ends and mix the same amount, adding it to whatever you have left in the applicator bottle.

26. Beginning at the nape of the neck, apply the bleach on the same 1/4-inch partings onto the middle lengths and ends on both the back sections (Figure 27).

27. Place a thick strip of cotton at the nape of the neck underneath the hair to protect the skin from the bleach.

28. Apply bleach to the middle lengths and ends of both front sections, taking the same 1/4-inch partings (Figure 28).

29. Place a wide strip of cotton underneath the hair at the temples to protect the skin on the face (Figure 29).

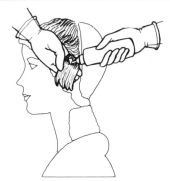

Figure 26

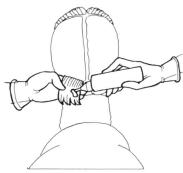

Figure 27

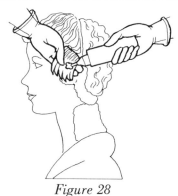

Figure 28

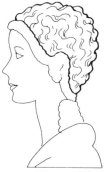

Figure 29

30. Your hair should now resemble a creamy blue soufflé. If you can see any of your hair, there is not enough bleach on it. (It is very important that you apply the bleach liberally to every section of the hair, and make certain that each parting is no more than 1/4-inch wide. This is because when ammonia and hydrogen peroxide are mixed together, oxidation occurs. Oxidation is basically an expansion of oxygen, which heats itself as it expands. If the partings are very close together, the bleach will touch, encouraging the self-heating process. If the bleach is sparsely applied, there will be tiny gaps into which air could pass. This would have a cooling effect, thereby reducing the effectiveness of the oxidation and creating an uneven result because the hair would lighten more in areas where it has been heavily applied.)

31. Allow the bleach to develop for thirty minutes.

32. Check a strand of hair by wiping it clean with a paper tissue to see if it's the same color from the scalp through to the ends of the hair. If it matches the test strand that you have previously done for bleach only, then shampoo. If it doesn't match your test strand, then allow another fifteen minutes and check again. Check every subsequent fifteen minutes until the correct level of yellow is achieved.

33. Once the correct yellow level has been arrived at, rinse the bleach thoroughly from your hair, paying special attention to the front part of the head where bleach is likely to be trapped under the hair.

34. Shampoo your hair, but **do not use a conditioner at this point.**

To Apply Toner

1. Put on your gloves.

2. Smear petroleum jelly around your hairline, neck and ears.

3. Gradually pour the toner onto your hair, massaging the color with the other hand until you have covered the entire head (Figure 30).

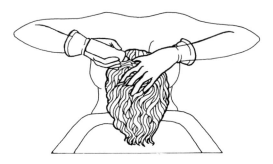

Figure 30

4. Place a strip of cotton over the petroleum jelly, around the hairline, ears and back of neck.

5. Cover the hair with the plastic cap provided and tighten it by pulling the front edge out in front of the face. Twist this edge so the cap fits tightly around the head and tuck the edge under the cap (Figure 31).

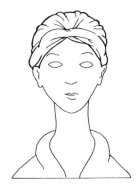

Figure 31

6. Allow the toner to develop for the full development time (between 20 and 30 minutes – check the manufacturer's instructions).

7. Remove the cap.

8. Add water to the toner and lather into its own shampoo (Figure 32).

To Finish

1. Condition your hair, either with the conditioner provided, or see Chapter 10.

2. Dry and style your hair.

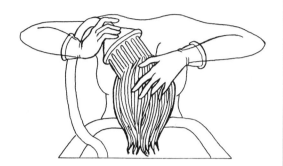

Figure 32

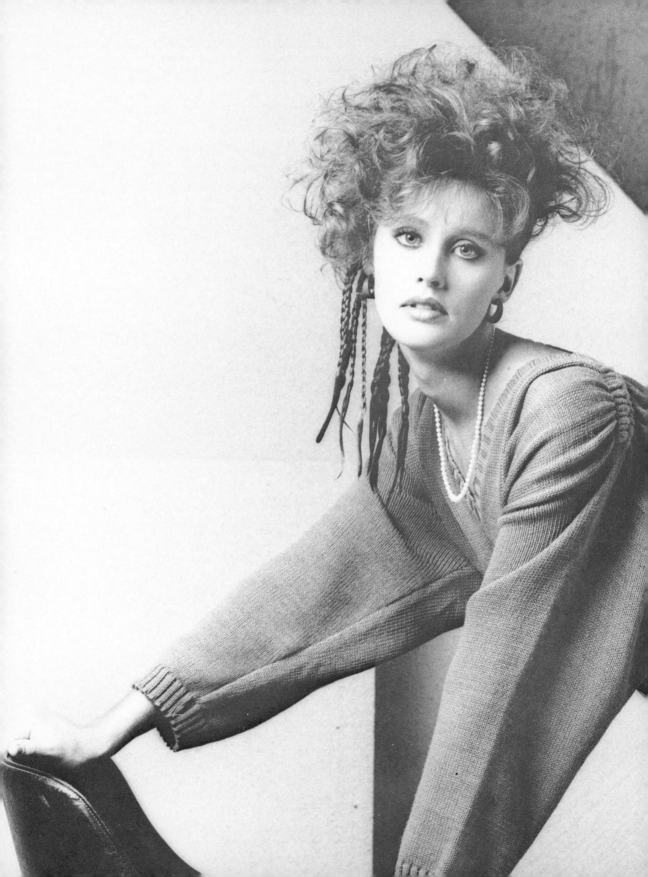

HIGHLIGHTS

Highlights

ADVANTAGES AND TECHNIQUES OF HIGHLIGHTING; WHEN TO HIGHLIGHT WITH BLEACH OR BLONDE; WHEN TO HIGHLIGHT WITH RED; WHEN TO HIGHLIGHT ON RED HAIR. HOW TO APPLY HIGHLIGHTS TO YOUR HAIR.

For many women, highlights provide the first adventure in coloring their hair. This is a very clever way of subtly changing your hair color, and about 80 percent of my coloring clientele is made up of people who have highlights.

So much can be achieved with highlights — so many different movements — that I will always use at least three different colors on one head of hair. By rearranging the natural highlights in hair I can change a mousy head into a dazzling display of color and tone.

ADVANTAGES OF HIGHLIGHTING

If highlighting is done correctly it has many advantages over any other form of color.

1. Low maintenance. Highlights only need to be redone every three to six months.

2. No noticeable regrowth. Many people want their hair to be more interesting than it is, but at the same time they don't want to be tied down to coloring their regrowth every month. There are others who can achieve the exact hair color they want without tinting — highlighting will do the job just as effectively by adding lightness or brightness. Highlighting is also the answer for those who are terrified to tint their hair in case they get bored with the color.

3. Will not adversely affect the condition of the hair because only some of the strands are being colored.

4. Can be used to blend in gray without completely changing the hair color.

5. Can emphasize the focal point of a hair cut.

6. Highlights can be used on any natural color of hair, including gray.

HIGHLIGHTING TECHNIQUES

Highlights were originally achieved by placing a rubber cap securely over the head and then pulling strands of hair through the tiny holes in the cap with a crochet hook. Bleach was then applied to the hair and was allowed to develop to a very pale blonde shade. Then the bleach was washed off the hair and a toner was applied according to the requirements of the client. After the toner had processed, the cap was removed and all the hair was shampooed. The client now had highlights.

Around 1960, the "frosting" technique, which is the precursor of the modern highlight tech-

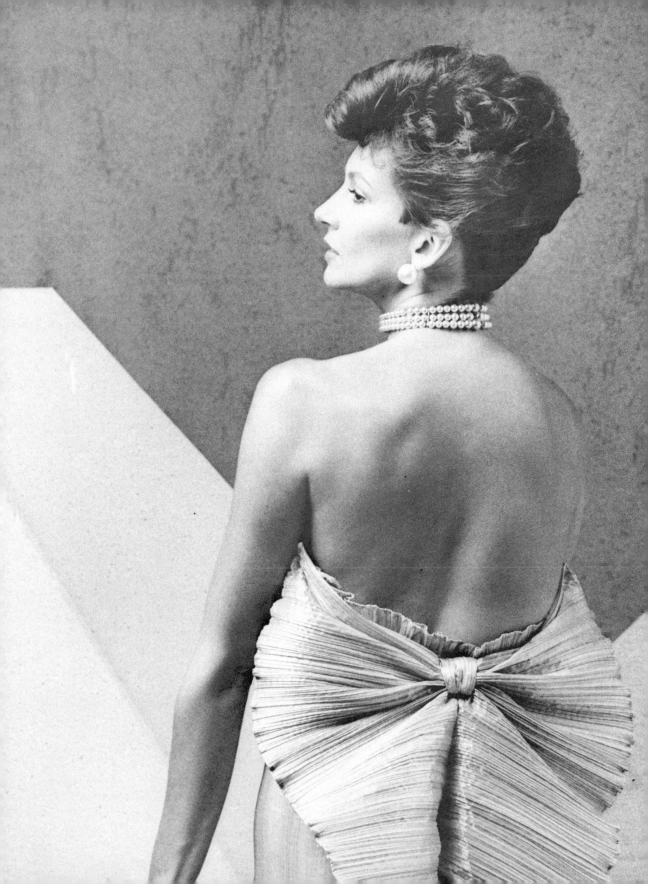

nique, was developed. Frosted hair was separated into 1/2-inch portions and one out of three were bleached, then wrapped in either cotton or foil. Nowadays, hair to be highlighted is sectioned into 1/4-inch partings and fine strands of hair are separated out from each section with the highlighting comb. Then bleach or color is applied and these sections are sealed into neat packages of foil or plastic wrap.

This technique is preferable to ''cap'' highlights mainly because the highlights look more natural. They are not in little clumps dispersed evenly through the whole head. Using this technique the highlights will also grow out more naturally, because there is not as much contrast with the natural color, and because the colorist has been consciously considering the growth pattern of the hair as well as the hairstyle when placing the highlights.

I have taught this technique to hairdressers throughout North America, most of whom were reluctant to stop using a cap. They have tried to persuade me that their clients prefer the cap method because it is faster and, therefore, less costly. Frankly, my own experience proves that this is simply not the case. Clients are invariably delighted when I tell them that I won't be using a cap, because it's painful and because they can see that the more painstaking technique improves the quality of their highlights. So my advice is to go to a salon where foil technique highlights are done. You won't regret the extra investment in time and money.

However, this chapter is devoted to teaching you how to do cap highlights for the following reasons:

1. There may not be a salon in your area where foil highlights are available.

2. You may not want to commit yourself to the cost.

3. You may just want to do it yourself. The kits for doing highlights at home use only the cap method.

WHEN TO HIGHLIGHT

1. If you want a subtle but definite change that lightens and/or brightens up your natural hair color.

2. If your hair is six inches in length or less.

THE HIGHLIGHT KIT

Manufacturers have now created products for the home market which are specifically designed for highlighting hair. Because the hair color does not touch the scalp in the highlighting process, they are able to make stronger colors with a greater capacity to lighten hair more than two levels. The colors are available in a limited range, but they still cover a wide spectrum.

A home highlighting kit will include the following items:

cap
crochet hook
small dish and spatula (to mix the product)
coloring product (permanent color + peroxide or bleach + peroxide)
plastic gloves
shampoo/conditioner
applicator brush

If these new highlighting kits are not yet available in your area, you will have to purchase your hair color separately (select the color according to the instructions described in Chapter 6). Then you will have to purchase a highlight cap either from your local drugstore or a beauty supply store. You will also need a crochet hook, size 12.

WHEN TO HIGHLIGHT WITH BLEACH

I recommend that, wherever possible, you use permanent color to highlight rather than bleach. However, if you are using bleach, it should only be used to highlight hair that is already blonde. Although bleach will eventually turn dark brown hair blonde, the combination of blonde highlights and dark brown hair is not very flattering.

Therefore, my rule of thumb for creating blonde highlights is that the natural color of the hair to be highlighted should be no darker than level 5, dark blonde. The level of blonde I wish to achieve determines whether a bleach or a tint is used. In the salon I rarely use bleach anymore because I can use a highlifting tint instead. But for home use, I suggest that if you wish your highlights to be more than three levels lighter than dark blonde, you use a bleach. (Using bleach to highlight is not as serious as bleaching the whole head because the bleach doesn't touch the scalp, and the regrowth is not as visible.)

Rule of Thumb: When highlighting with bleach, you should make certain that there is at least 1/2-inch between the holes in the highlight cap. I do not advise that you re-highlight your hair until the original highlights grow out. The greater distance between the highlights means that the regrowth will not be as visible. If the holes in your cap appear in greater frequency, don't use all of them. Take a brightly colored pencil and circle those holes that you wish to use.

WHEN TO HIGHLIGHT WITH BLONDE TINT

The highlight kits contain blonde tints which are preferable to using bleach to highlight on blonde hair. To highlight with these blonde tints, your natural color should be at least a level 5, dark blonde. Moreover, you will see that you have two options within the blonde range. You can add either gold tones or ash tones, but if you do, these should already be in your hair. In the not too distant future, a product should be available which will allow you to achieve a two- or three-tone effect. In the meantime you can invent your own. Just buy three different blonde tints: an ash blonde, a golden blonde and an orange blonde. Then carefully apply each blonde tone in lines across the cap, repeating the rotation as often as possible. The result will be multicolored blonde tones (Figure 33).

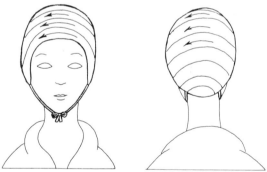

Figure 33

WHEN TO HIGHLIGHT WITH RED

Kits for adding red or orange highlights (around the level of medium blonde) are now on the market. The reds won't lighten but they will add color. Therefore, they should be used on hair that is any color of brown, especially medium or dark brown. If you really want to become creative you could add dramatic red highlights to your dark blonde hair. Use the kit that contains the orange-red highlights.

If you want to create multicolored red tones, buy three separate tints in the chestnut tones: a deep red, copper and gold. Start from the base of the cap and cover the first two inches with red. Then, working toward the crown, cover the next two inches with copper and the remainder with the gold color. This gives the impression that the hair is darker around the hairline, lightening gradually as it reaches the crown (Figure 34).

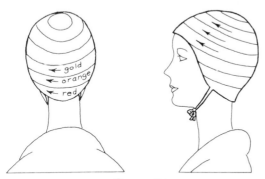

Figure 34

WHEN TO HIGHLIGHT ON RED HAIR

Sometimes as redheads reach their mid-thirties a lot of the sparkle of their red disappears. This is an ideal time to add red highlights to your hair.

Rule of Thumb: When highlighting red hair, use the alternative red to that which is dominant in your hair. For example, if your hair is naturally medium copper blonde, I would rekindle that color with flame red blonde highlights. As you can see from the color chart (see page 26), it is found on the same level (level 6) as your natural color but under a different tone.

HOW TO HIGHLIGHT YOUR HAIR

What You Need

highlighting kit (see page 86)
or
highlighting cap
crochet hook, size 12
small dish and spatula (to mix the product) or applicator bottle(s)
permanent color(s) or bleach + peroxide
applicator brush
plastic gloves
plastic wrap
shampoo and conditioner
baby powder
comb
paper tissues

To Prepare

1. At least 48 hours before highlighting your hair, give yourself a sensitivity test (if you are using permanent color) and do a strand test (or tests, if more than one color is to be used). See pages 41 and 42.

2. In the bathroom or kitchen, lay out everything you will need in front of you.

3. Put on your gloves.

4. Dust the inside of the cap with baby powder.

5. Comb your hair in the basic shape of your hairstyle, but make sure that the hair nearest the hairline is combed slightly away to reveal the hairline. If you have a part in your hair, make sure it is well revealed.

6. Pull the cap onto your head, trying not to disturb the way you have combed your hair.

To Highlight

1. Starting at the hairline, take the hook and gently press it through the holes in the cap. As the hook touches the scalp, pull the hair attached to the hook through the hole. Make sure that you pull no more than twenty strands of hair through each hole (Figure 35).

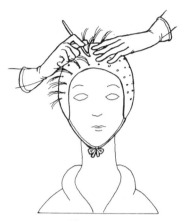

Figure 35

2. Continue pulling hair through the holes along all the hairline.

3. Proceed to the row 1/2-inch back from the first row and repeat the procedure.

4. Continue doing this in rows until you have covered all the cap.

5. For highlights with bleach, pour the bleach into the dish provided. Add peroxide and mix with the spatula. For highlights with color, mix the color(s) in the applicator bottle(s) provided.

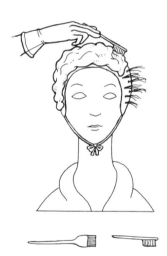

Figure 36

6. Liberally apply color or bleach with the applicator brush to all the exposed strands of hair (Figure 36).

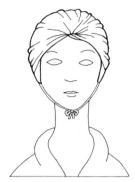

Figure 37

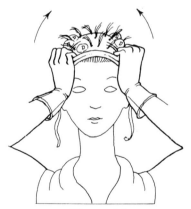

Figure 38

7. If a plastic cap is provided, cover the color or bleach with it (Figure 37). This will keep the scalp warm. Oxidation will take place and ensure the correct target color. If a plastic cap is not provided, wrap plastic wrap over your head to achieve the same result.

8. Allow the color or bleach to develop for the time already determined by the strand test(s).

9. Check a strand of hair by wiping it clean with a paper tissue to see if it's the same color as the test strand.

10. If it is not an even color, cover again with the plastic cap or plastic wrap and check again after 10 minutes. When it *is* an even color, rinse the bleach or color off the hair but **leave the highlighting cap on the head.** Add shampoo to the highlighted hair.

11. Now, gently lift the cap up and away from your head (Figure 38). The shampoo will have lubricated the hair, allowing it to slide through the holes painlessly.

To Finish

1. Shampoo the whole head.

2. Condition with the conditioner provided, or see Chapter 10.

3. Dry and style your hair.

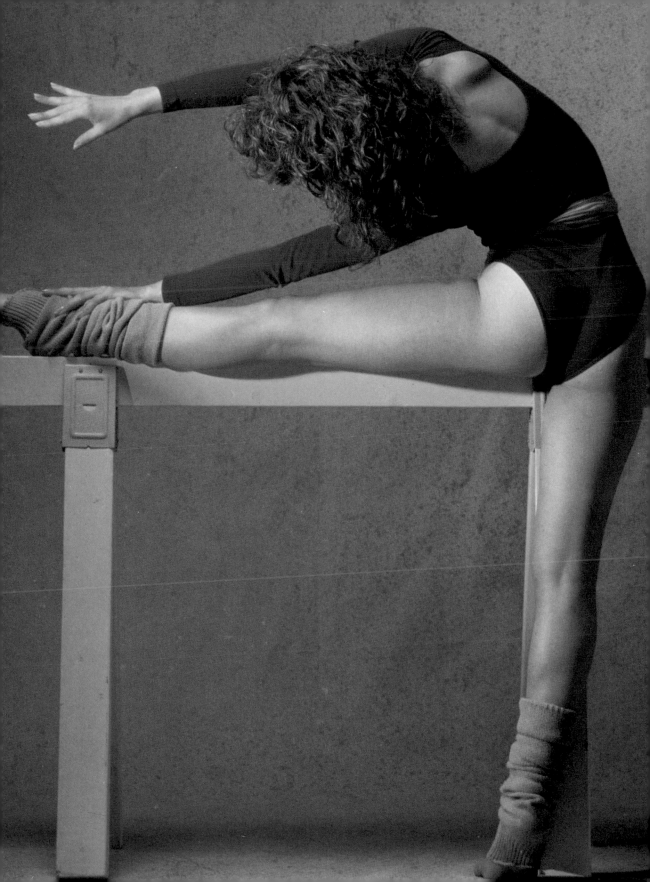

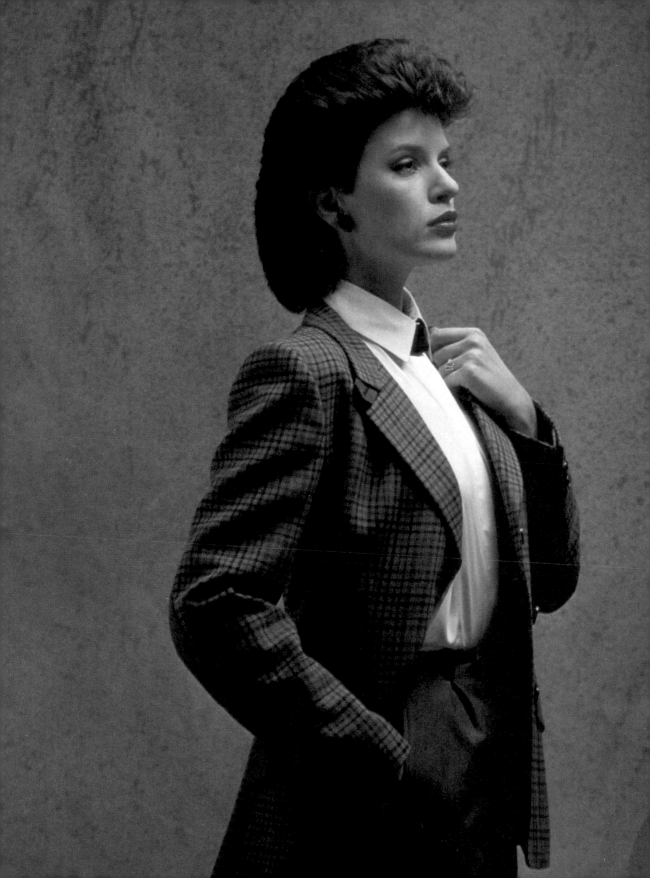

HENNA

HENNA

WHAT IT IS AND WHAT IT WILL DO; WHEN NOT TO USE HENNA. HOW TO CHOOSE THE CORRECT HENNA COLOR AND APPLY IT.

In the 1970's I worked in a London salon called Molton Brown. What I learned there still influences how I feel about hair color and hair in general. I firmly believe that one should try to keep hair in the best possible condition. Chemical work is most successful on top-quality hair. As well, I believe that hair color is most interesting when it appears to be natural.

This is the legacy passed on to me by the owner of that salon. His name is Michael Collis and he has always been concerned about creating natural-looking hairstyles — he was, for instance, the innovator of finger-drying hair. Because we were very interested in experimenting with natural products, we developed our own camomile and rosemary shampoos, as well as natural hair conditioners and natural hair colors.

We also used a great deal of henna, and in the process I learned how to achieve some excellent results with that product. For instance, I discovered that by mixing beetroot with red henna I could create a marvellous burgundy color. Nowadays, henna has declined in popularity along with the whole earth movement that spawned its boom. But it's still a useful product for coloring hair, particularly if you are allergic to chemical hair colors. The only thing you can be allergic to in henna is the powder itself. Moreover, you will only react as to an irritant, like hay fever. It should not produce a serious reaction.

What Henna Is

Henna is a natural hair color. It is derived from the leaf of a plant that belongs to the privet family which grows throughout Asia and north Africa. Women have used it for centuries as a hair color and make-up as well as for its medicinal value. Not only does henna condition, color and strengthen the hair, giving it a luxurious shine, it also heals sores, burns and skin irritations.

In the past, henna was primarily used as a conditioner. Nowadays, though, we use it more for its coloring properties, as we have access to superior products for conditioning hair.

Not all henna is of uniform quality. Basically, the richer the soil in which the henna plant grows, the better the henna. Moreover, henna improves as one travels east. In Morocco, henna grows in arid soil, therefore, it's tough and yields a weak, yellow-gold color. In Asia, Iran, Israel and Egypt, the soil in which the henna is cultivated is far richer, giving us a deep orange. In India the soil is richer still and produces the deep henna red.

Hairdressers buy henna already packaged from beauty supply stores, where it has arrived already blended into different warm tones. Using henna we can produce colors ranging from gold to black. To produce the different tones of brown or black, the following natural dyes are blended with henna:

Indigo: Indigo is the oldest and most widely used dye in history. Legend has it that the prophet Mohammed dyed his beard black using the indigo plant. Indigo has a blue/violet tone, and when it is mixed with henna a very dark brown/black color results.

Vashma: The vashma plant is always blended with ground castor beans (karchak) before being added to henna. The final effect is a dark brown or ash brown.

Wode: The dye from this plant has been used for centuries in the Middle East and in Britain. It is pale blue in color and was used particularly for dying clothes and in makeup. Blonde women used to rinse their hair with wode to lessen the yellow tinge that often occurs with age. Wode combines with pale henna to create soft ash blonde effects.

Lote: The leaves of the lote tree have blue-green properties and they combine with henna to create soft iridescent browns.

Sadr: The sadr tree has very pale leaves that produce a pale ash to colorless tone. The leaves contain the best natural astringent for controlling oily hair. When mixed with henna leaves that have been stripped of their veins, sadr produces neutral henna. This is the colorless henna that is used for conditioning only.

Henna Shade	Contents
red henna	henna
brown henna	henna, lote, wode
golden henna	henna, sadr
chestnut henna	henna, wode
dark warm brown henna	henna, karchack, vashma
black henna	henna, vashma, karchack, indigo
neutral henna	neutral henna, sadr

What Henna Will Do

The henna leaf contains a substance known as Lawsonia which both colors and conditions hair. This substance works both by penetrating the hair and by coating and staining the hair. By adding warm water to henna, you create a paste which warms and softens the hair, making it receptive to the color. You can see an immediate improvement in the condition of the hair as the Lawsonia works itself into the hair, coloring and conditioning simultaneously.

Rule of Thumb: With the exception of golden or neutral henna, henna should only be used on brown hair to add color. It will not make hair lighter. Neutral henna will condition hair, but in my opinion you'll achieve much better results with a protein pack (see Chapter 10).

WHEN NOT TO USE HENNA

1. **On permed hair.** Henna can stretch the curl or wave and, therefore, make the perm relax too much.

2. **Over a tint.** Henna tends to dehydrate the hair over a period of time. It will make a tint fade more quickly and you could end up with the regrowth from your henna being a lighter color than your natural hair color. Henna should also not be mixed with a permanent hair color, bleach and/or hydrogen peroxide.

3. **Red henna should not be used on blondes.** The hair would become a bright red.

4. **On gray hair.** Because the pigments in henna are so strong, they would tint white hair either brilliant red or orange, or black, depending upon the color used.

Rule of Thumb: I would strongly recommend that only those of you with natural color levels 1-4 apply henna at home. For those with natural color levels 5-9, I would recommend that henna only be applied by your hairdresser.

HENNA COLORS AND DEVELOPMENT TIMES

Henna Color	Natural Color								
	Black (1)	Dark Brown (2)	Medium Brown (3)	Light Brown (4)	Dark Blonde (5)	Medium Blonde (6)	Light Blonde (7)	Very Light Blonde (8)	Extra Light Blonde (9)
Natural Red	shine 60 minutes	dark red brown highlights 2 hours	deep red brown 2 hours	light red brown 60 minutes	dark red blonde 20 minutes	1/2 neutral + 1/2 natural red = medium red blonde 20 minutes	3/4 neutral + 1/4 natural red = light red blonde 15 minutes		
Black	jet black 2 hours	deep black 90 minutes	black 90 minutes	darkest brown 80 minutes					
Dark Warm Brown	shine 60 minutes	rich dark brown 2 hours	rich medium brown 90 minutes	rich light brown 60 minutes	dark warm blonde 40 minutes	medium warm blonde 30 minutes	1/2 dark warm brown + 1/2 neutral = light warm blonde 20 minutes		
Chestnut Brown	shine 60 minutes	shine 60 minutes	chestnut brown 80 minutes	light chestnut brown 60 minutes	warm chestnut 40 minutes	chestnut blonde 30 minutes			
Brown	shine 60 minutes	shine 60 minutes	copper brown 90 minutes	light copper brown 60 minutes	rich copper blonde 40 minutes	bright copper 40 minutes			
Golden	shine 60 minutes	shine 60 minutes	soft golden brown 90 minutes	light golden brown 60 minutes	dark golden blonde 40 minutes	golden blonde 30 minutes	1/2 golden + 1/2 neutral = light golden blonde 30 minutes	1/4 golden + 3/4 neutral = light gold 30 minutes	

Note: The longer henna is left on the hair *over* these suggested times, the brighter the result will be.
Note: If you have a hood dryer at home, you could use it to reduce the time required to develop the henna. The addition of heat will cut the development time in half.

HOW TO APPLY HENNA

What You Need

henna

mixing bowl

wooden spoon

petroleum jelly

piece of aluminum foil, 12 inches by 30 inches

pair of surgical gloves

strips of cotton batting

towels

newspapers to cover the floor

shampoo

To Prepare

1. Select an appropriate color using the chart on page 96. (The contents of a packet of henna is enough to cover hair up to 8 inches in length. If your hair is longer you will need to purchase more than one packet.)

2. Do a strand test to make certain that the color you have selected will produce the desired results. Mix up a very small amount of henna (using hot water to form a paste). Apply it to about twenty strands of hair cut from the nape of the neck. Wrap the hair in aluminum foil and let it process for the required amount of time.

3. Completely cover the floor area where you will be applying the henna to your hair with newspaper. It is a very messy procedure; the henna crumbles easily and it can stain your floor.

4. Put on your gloves.

5. Place the desired quantity of henna in a mixing bowl.

6. Gradually add hot water from the tap, mixing with the spoon until you have a smooth paste.

7. Apply a generous amount of petroleum jelly around your hairline and on the back of your neck and ears. (If you do not do this, you will have an orange face and neck for days.)

To Henna

1. Divide your hair into four sections by taking one parting from ear to ear and another from the center of the forehead to the nape of the neck (Figure 39).

2. Start applying henna to the two back sections first. With the index finger, take a parting of approximately 1-1/2 inches. Hold the remaining hair in that section away with the other hand.

3. Scoop a sufficient amount of henna and pat it on that first small section (Figure 40). Using the fingers, work it through all that hair from scalp to ends.

4. Twist that hennaed piece of hair into a ringlet (Figure 41).

5. Proceed with the next small section in the same way. When you have finished the first back area, twist all the single ringlets together and then start applying henna to the second back area.

6. When the final back section is completed you can begin on the front two sections. Once again, take 1-1/2-inch partings with the index finger, but start at the temple and work in a diagonal pattern toward the centre of the crown, making sure that each separate parting has been twisted into individual ringlets as you proceed.

7. Twist the individual ringlets into one large one.

8. Proceed with the final quarter, as above.

9. Now all the hair is covered with henna and twisted into four separate bunches. (This twisting of the hair ensures a complete and even distribution of henna along each hair.) Join the four bunches together. First take the two back pieces and lift up to the crown, twisting

simultaneously. Do the same with the two front pieces. As they meet at the top of the crown, twist all four together. The hair will lock and stay together on the crown (Figure 42).

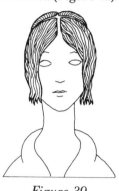

Figure 39

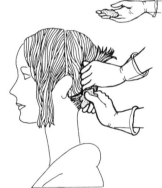

Figure 40

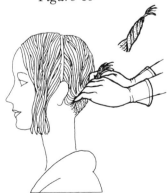

Figure 41

10. Take a strip of cotton and place it on top of the petroleum jelly around the hairline (Figure 43).

11. Take a sheet of aluminum foil and fold the edges over 1/2 inch. (This is to make certain that the sharp edges won't cut you.)

12. Wrap the foil around your head and scrunch it to the top of your head, pressing firmly so that it fits tightly over the hair. It should seal like a secure aluminum cap covering the head (Figure 44).

13. Allow the henna to develop for the required amount of time suggested on the chart (page 96). The longer the henna is left on **over** these times, the brighter the result will be. This is all you have to do until it's time to shampoo the henna off. To make sure you don't tread bits of henna through the house, this is a good time to clean up. (If you do stain any surfaces with henna, rinse them with shampoo immediately. The longer the henna sits, the more stubborn the stain. Eventually, though, it will wash off.)

To Finish

1. When the time to shampoo has arrived, go to your bathroom and, leaning over the tub, remove the foil. This way any dry pieces of henna will fall into the bath and not onto the floor.

2. Rinse your hair in warm water for at least 10 minutes to remove all the henna. If you are standing under the shower, be sure to rinse your hair well in the nape of your neck because the henna can get trapped under the hair. If you are leaning over a sink or bath, the weight of your hair will be over your face, so make sure no henna is trapped under that part of your hair.

3. Shampoo your hair with your regular shampoo and then rinse very thoroughly again. Your hair should not need any conditioner as the henna has

done that job for you. If your hair still feels gritty, shampoo again and comb the shampoo through before rinsing.

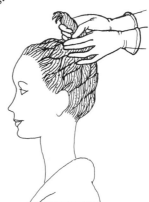

Figure 42

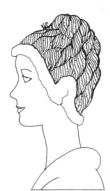

Figure 43

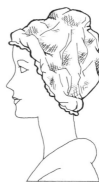

Figure 44

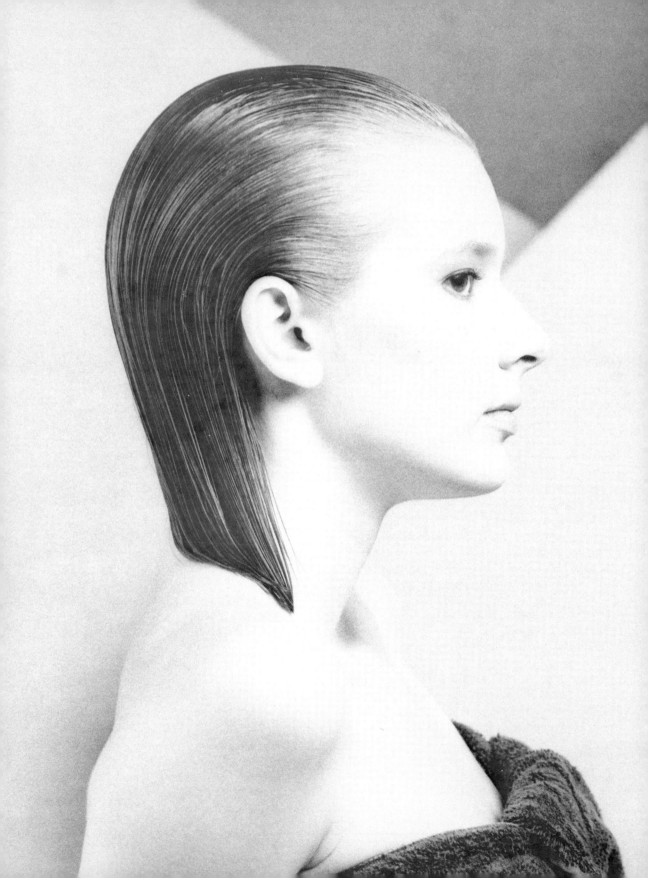

HOW TO CARE FOR YOUR HAIR

HOW TO CARE FOR YOUR HAIR

PROTEIN-BASED HAIR CARE PRODUCTS: SHAMPOO, MOISTURIZER, PROTEIN-RINSE AND PROTEIN PACK; CARING FOR OILY, NORMAL AND DRY HAIR. HOW TO BRUSH AND COMB YOUR HAIR AND WHEN TO HAVE YOUR HAIR CUT.

When I was working in London in 1969, I had a client in her late seventies who had one of the most beautiful heads of hair I have ever seen. It was waist length and gray and silkily luxurious. I softened it with a silver ash semipermanent color.

Her hair was so beautiful because she took excellent care of it. Every morning and night she brushed it sixty-five times, so although she used only a simple green soap shampoo, she never needed a conditioner or oil treatment – the brushing provided enough scalp stimulation. Moreover, she was extremely fit because she walked at least five miles every single day. She had been doing this since childhood, just as she had been faithfully following a sensible balanced diet.

Not only is this dear lady one in a million, she is also a symbol of the vanishing lives we used to lead. When everything was much more simple, we did have time to pamper ourselves at home. We also ate fresher, more natural foods. So in those days, we could keep our hair in excellent condition just by brushing it regularly and using a basic shampoo.

Nowadays, most of us don't follow a balanced diet, keep as fit as we should or even have time to brush our hair sixty-five times morning and night. We're also much more inclined to use chemicals on our hair, either coloring it, perming it or frequently doing both. We use hot rollers or curling irons, or we blow dry it, tugging at tangles until they end up in the comb or the brush. In short, we don't take very good care of our hair.

And in some cases, who can really blame us? Consider, for instance, that the number of women in the work force has risen dramatically in the last decade. A woman who is juggling the often-conflicting demands of a home life and a career simply doesn't have time to pamper herself. The problem is that because she is in the public eye so much, her appearance is even more important than it used to be.

These changes have influenced the way we look at hair. A woman who has a full-time career and a family, who possibly works out three times a week, or jogs several miles a day to keep fit, does not want a hairstyle that needs to be set in rollers, baked under a dryer, backcombed and sprayed with lacquer so it won't move for a week. She wants to be able to shampoo her hair often, and to dry it quickly. She also wants a style that is both attractive and sexy.

There are few of us, I think, who would trade the active and busy lives we lead today for the more restricted ones of the past. Even so, contemporary lifestyles place an enormous amount of stress on our bodies and our hair. Just as we take vitamin pills to supply our bodies with nutrients that our fast-food diets might not provide, so should we think about feeding our hair with the protein it needs to remain healthy and shiny. Fortunately, technology has provided us with the means to do this.

In the past decade, manufacturers have developed a wide range of new hair-care products. Hair, as you may know, is composed of protein. Thus chemists have found a way to make protein with a molecular structure so small that it can penetrate into the hair, and strengthen and improve it. We now have products containing "micronized protein." I think they're indispensible in caring for your hair.

Let me explain. The basic shampoos of the past cleaned the hair, but they left it feeling very dry. So in those days we conditioned hair with either a lanolin or emulsified wax base or balsam, which left the hair feeling either very soft and "flyaway,"

or heavy and dull. So too, the deep treatments of hot oil which were shampooed out of the hair, left it feeling just as dry as it had been before the so-called treatment.

But the new products containing micronized protein will not only clean, they will actually repair less-than-perfect hair, because they do more than remain on the surface of the hair. Their tiny molecular structure allows them to be taken into the hair where they can actually improve its quality. (Although some "natural" hair care products are good, in my opinion they are generally not as effective as the new shampoos and conditioners based on micronized protein.)

How can you identify these products? There's a very simple rule: with a very few exceptions they are only available in beauty salons. However, there are a few lines that are available elsewhere, and the rule of thumb to follow is that if you can buy the product in a beauty salon, you can buy it wherever it's for sale.

You will recognize the new protein-based lines by the range of products they include: shampoo, moisturizer, possibly a protein rinse and always a protein pack. (When using these products always stick to the same line. Don't use one manufacturer's shampoo, another's moisturizer and a third's protein pack. These products are scientifically formulated to produce a particular result. That is, they are chemically balanced like a long equation: $A + B + C = X$. If any one of those components is changed, the result will not be as the manufacturers predicted.)

PROTEIN-BASED HAIR CARE PRODUCTS

1. **Shampoo:** The type of shampoo, whether it's for normal, dry, chemically-treated or oily hair should be determined by your own hair.

2. **Moisturizer:** Moisturizers contain moisture proteins which are absorbed into the hair. They contain no oil, or anything that tends to make hair feel greasy, and in certain instances they can be supplemented with a protein rinse. A moisturizer should be used after every shampoo because your hair, like your skin, naturally loses a certain amount of its own natural moisture when it's washed. A moisturizer will also soften the hair and therefore improve its feel. (A moisturizer is not a cream rinse. A cream rinse will not improve the condition of your hair. It will only make it softer and easier to comb.)

3. **Protein rinse:** This product seals the cuticle and protects the inside of the hair (the cortex), thereby forming a protective barrier. A protein rinse is either sprayed into the hair or applied from the bottle. Some hairdressers will recommend that, depending upon your hair type, you substitute the protein rinse for the moisturizer after every shampoo.

4. **Protein pack:** This is an *intensified* protein hair treatment which supplies both the cortex and the cuticle with all the protein they require. Depending upon the condition and quality of the hair, it will last for about eight shampoos. It is the basis for great conditioned hair.

After the hair has been shampooed, the contents of the pack are liberally dispersed throughout the hair. It is combed through from the hairline, straight back, unless you have long hair, in which case it should be combed toward the crown where the hair is then fixed with a plastic clip.

The only heat I like to use with a protein pack is the natural heat of the head. Wrap plastic wrap over the hair to seal in the natural warmth and leave for the required amount of time. Although most manufacturers will recommend that the pack be left on for five minutes, you can extend that up to twenty minutes. At that point, your hair will have absorbed all the protein that it is capable of absorbing and it is pointless to leave the pack on any longer. The pack is then rinsed off and the hair is dried.

You should not use a protein pack on freshly colored hair. Hair that has just been colored is slightly porous. Therefore, as the pack treatment is absorbed into the hair some of the color pigments will attach themselves to some of the protein. The hair will only absorb a certain amount of protein so that when the pack is rinsed out of the hair, it may take some of the color with it, and the color will fade.

Even if you are applying protein packs regularly at home, I recommend that you also have an intensified salon protein treatment every six to eight weeks, as long as the treatment does not coincide with technical work such as coloring.

CARING FOR OILY HAIR

Contrary to conventional wisdom, it is very rare these days for people to have excessively oily hair. Excessively oily hair is hair that becomes oily within twenty-four hours of being washed. Normal, healthy hair will become oily within two to three days of being shampooed.

If your hair does qualify as oily, you should make a list of the things that you eat every day and consult a dietician. Your glands are producing too much sebum and a dietician may be able to tell you how to correct this.

If your oily hair is washed every day, the ends are likely dry. So after you have shampooed your hair (ideally with shampoo made for oily hair), it will probably feel very dry and rather hard. Therefore, you will need to use a moisturizer to moisturize just

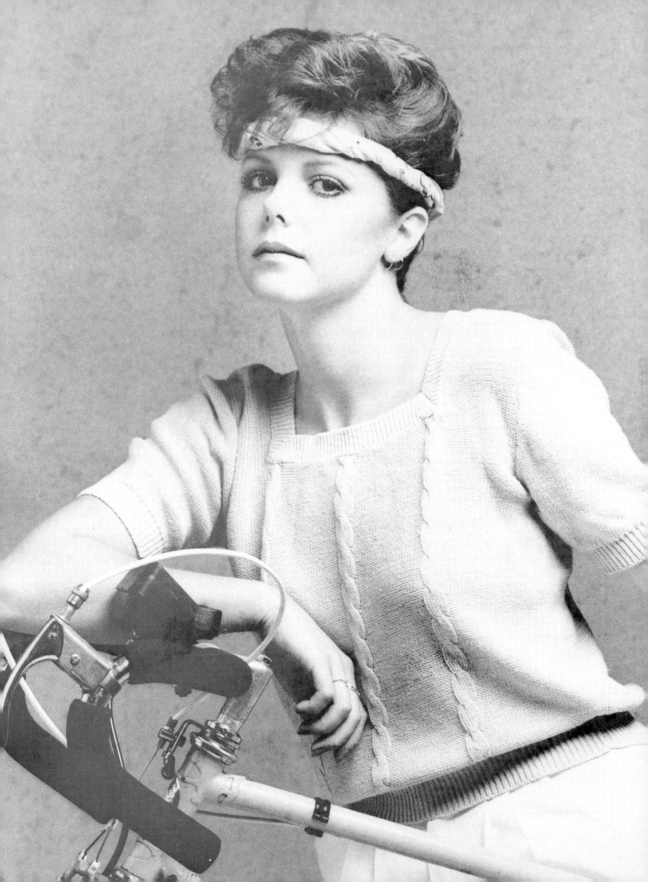

the ends of the hair. In fact, if you have not been using a moisturizer, this may help to explain why your hair is so oily. The oil glands are over-producing to reach the dry ends of your hair.

If your hair is excessively oily, you should be using a protein rinse on top of a moisturizer. This will help the hair to retain moisture and as the moisture content of the ends improves, you should notice (over a period of four to six weeks) that your glands are not producing as much sebum.

When you see a noticeable improvement in your hair, try to shampoo every second day using the same three products. You should see a further improvement. Then change to a shampoo for normal hair. Continue with moisturizer and protein rinse until you are convinced that after two or three days your hair is still in excellent condition. Then you can begin to *alternate* between using a moisturizer and a protein rinse after every shampoo. After every eight shampoos your should use a protein pack. This will help to speed up the reconditioning of the ends.

CARING FOR NORMAL HAIR

If your hair has **not** been chemically treated with either a permanent wave, semipermanent color, tint or a bleach or highlights; if it only needs to be shampooed every second or third day; if you don't need a conditioner of some sort to detangle it after a shampoo; if it has a wonderful shine when you dry it; then your hair is considered normal.

However, the word "normal" is a misnomer because I know of very few people to whom the above description would apply. But for the purposes of choosing a hair care regimen, if your hair is not excessively dry or excessively oily, even if it is chemically treated, you can consider it to be "normal."

If your hair is "normal" you should use a shampoo for normal hair, and a moisturizer each time you shampoo. You should also follow up with the protein rinse if your hair has been chemically treated. After every eight shampoos, replace the moisturizer and protein rinse with a protein pack treatment.

CARING FOR DRY HAIR

Dry hair is hair that is moisture-starved. This can result from using a poor-quality shampoo. I remember a client I once had in London, who complained that the color of her hair was fading and that it was in terrible condition. I wasn't surprised when I learned that she washed her hair with dishwashing detergent. "If it's good enough for my dishes, it's good enough for my hair," she said. I had to explain to her that the harshness of this detergent was responsible for the excessive dryness of her hair. Once she understood, she switched to better shampoo and the quality of her hair improved dramatically.

Excessive exposure to the sun, sea or wind can also damage your hair, as can swimming in a chlorinated pool or chemical work such as permanent waves, tints, bleaches, highlights, etc. The greater the combination of these elements on your hair, the greater the potential for damage and dryness. (If your hair has been tinted or bleached, swimming in a chlorinated pool can remove some of the hair color and make your hair very dry. Blondes and redheads should be especially cautious because the chlorine can actually cause the hair to change color.)

Moisturizing shampoo is the only shampoo which contains moisture protein. It is absorbed into the hair by massaging the hair and the scalp as you shampoo. If you have dry hair, you will obviously have to devote more effort to improving its condition than you would with the other types.

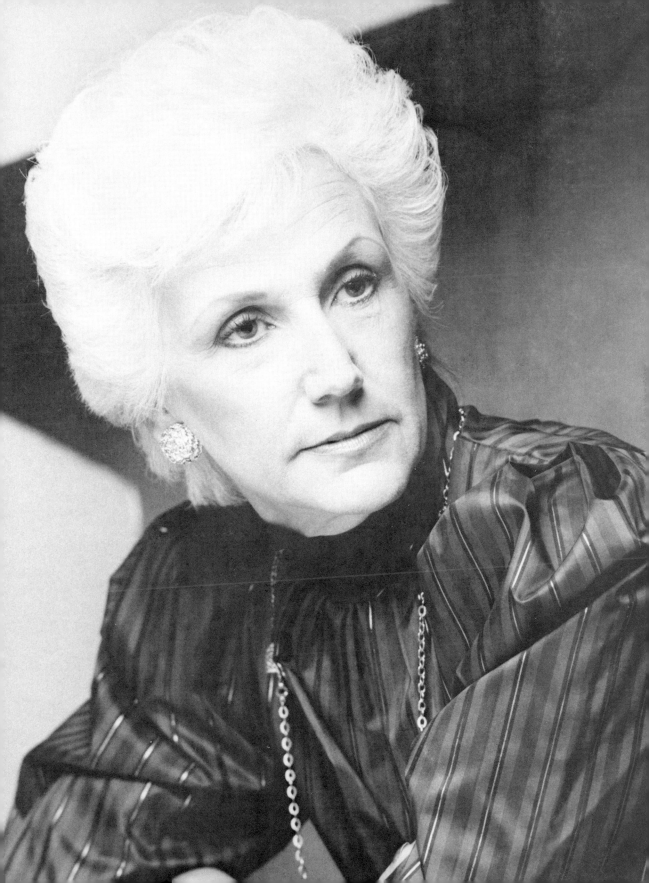

Every time you shampoo you will need to use a moisturizer **and** a protein rinse. To begin with, I suggest that you use a protein pack once a week or after three shampoos. As the condition of your hair improves (it will take about six weeks for you to notice a difference), you can reduce the number of pack treatments to every eight shampoos. However, I strongly suggest that while hair is being chemically treated or exposed to the sun that you continue using the other three products every time you shampoo.

HOW TO COMB YOUR HAIR

If your hair is damaged, you can actually help to improve its quality by combing it properly. Even if your hair is in good condition, you can increase its chance of remaining so by combing it in the correct manner.

First, never try to comb wet hair with anything except a wide-tooth comb. Taking the comb, you should start combing the hair from the nape of the neck. Begin at the ends and gradually work toward the hair nearest the scalp, losening each tangle as your proceed. You will find, in fact, that it will comb out quite easily, quickly and painlessly, and you will not be subjecting your hair to the kind of ruthless tugging that can cause it to split and break.

HOW TO BRUSH YOUR HAIR

You should **never** use a brush to remove tangles in your hair. A wide-tooth comb is far more effective. However, it is not an old wives' tale that brushing the hair improves its health. It stimulates the blood vessels of the scalp and helps us to have naturally healthy, shiny hair. Use a natural bristle brush and start by brushing the hair at the nape of the neck, lifting most of the hair up with your other hand. As you continue brushing, allow layers of hair to fall, gradually working your way up to the crown.

WHEN TO CUT YOUR HAIR

You will proabaly need to have your hair trimmed every four to six weeks in order for it to maintain its proper shape and bounce. This is true even if you are trying to grow out your hair. Frequent trims will help to keep it looking attractive.

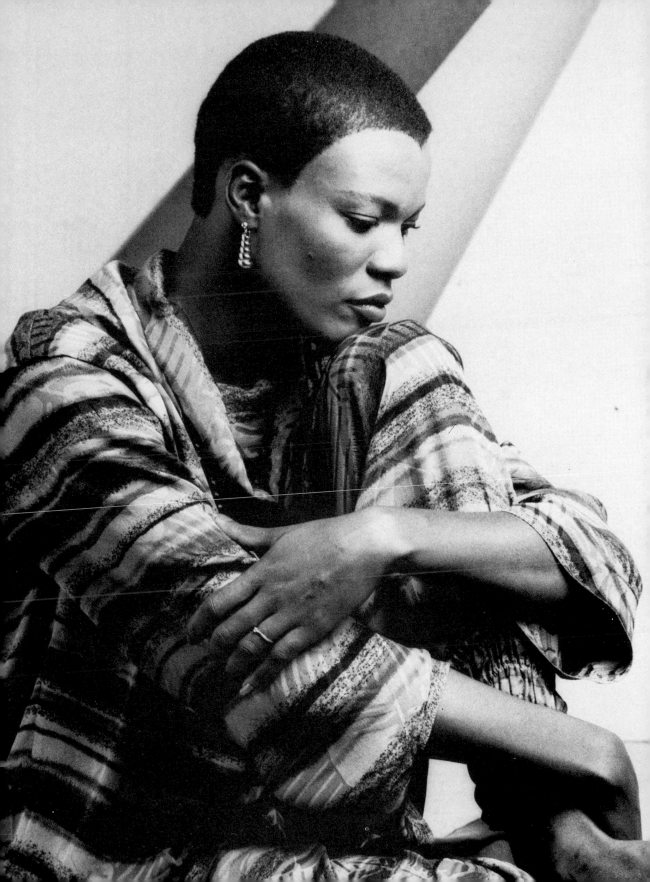

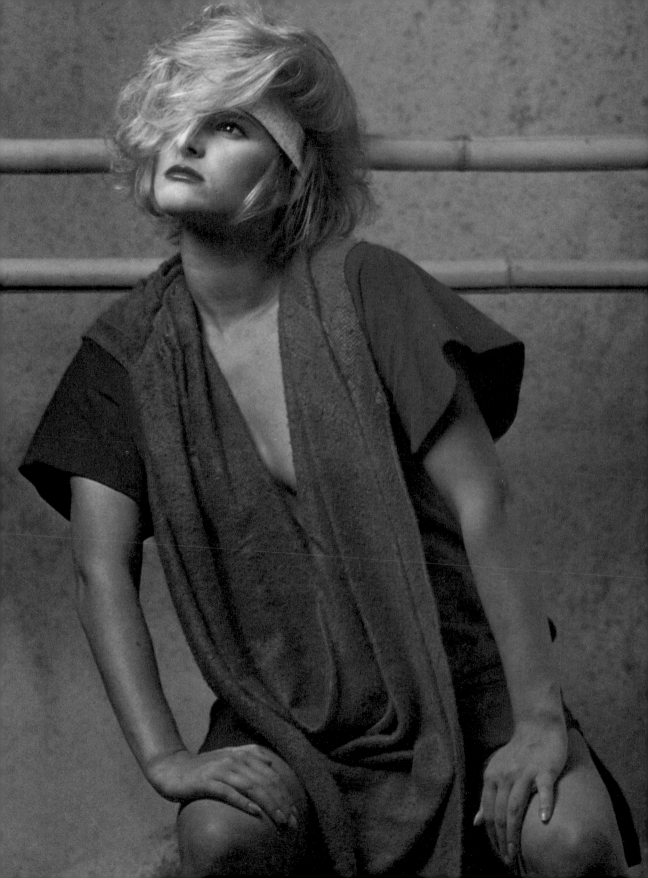

What only your hairdresser can do for you

WHAT ONLY YOUR HAIRDRESSER CAN DO FOR YOU

HOW TO RECOGNIZE A GOOD SALON AND WHAT TO LOOK FOR IN A COLOR TECHNICIAN. THINGS ONLY YOUR HAIRDRESSER SHOULD DO FOR YOU: BLEACHING, COLOR CORRECTION, RETURNING TO YOUR NATURAL COLOR FROM ARTIFICIAL BLONDE, RETURNING TO GRAY, COLOR PLUS A PERMANENT WAVE.

From time to time, a client will move to another city and she will ask me if I can recommend a good hairdresser in her new area. Sometimes I can and my job is easy. I will also pass along the formula for the color I have been using on her hair.

But in many cases, I know no one whom I can recommend, so often clients end up asking me for advice on how to recognize a good salon. Unfortunately, there is no foolproof method, but here are some guidelines.

HOW TO RECOGNIZE A GOOD SALON

If you are new to a city, it's a good idea to make a point of looking at the women you see on the street. When you see one with hair that you really like, just ask her where she has it done. No one minds receiving a compliment, so your chances of getting the name of a salon are very good. Phone that salon and make an appointment for a consultation. This should be *free*.

I realize that going to a new salon for a hair cut can be a nerve-racking experience. If you are having your hair colored or permed, it may be truly terrifying. Therefore, it is your right to ask as many questions as it will take to make you feel confident that you are placing yourself in good hands.

If you live in a city, I would strongly recommend that you only go to a salon that has a technician — a hairdresser who specializes in color and permanent waves.

WHAT TO LOOK FOR IN A TECHNICIAN

When asssessing a client's hair, a technician should use daylight whenever possible. Or the salon should have a lighting system that resembles daylight. A good color technician should ask whether you are satisfied with the color you have. If so, he should ask whether you have your formula with you. If you do, he should be able to repeat it exactly.

If you haven't brought your formula, the technician should immediately look at the color of your roots and then at the color of the rest of your hair. If this does not happen, ask him what he is going to use and how he arrived at that decision. Having determined your natural color using the method described in Chapter 3, you should be able to tell whether or not the technician knows what he is talking about.

Ask how they apply the color. Do they use an applicator bottle or a brush? If they use an applicator bottle, give them one strike against. So too, with highlights. A good salon will do highlights with plastic wrap or aluminum foil. They will not use a highlight cap.

Look at the other clients, checking to see whether their color has been applied messily or neatly. Is there any color on the neck or the face? Is there a barrier cream around the hairline? Does the technican wear gloves? If the answers to all these questions are positive, then it's likely that you're in good hands.

If you are not living in a city big enough to have salons with their own color technician, then you will have to place yourself in the hands of the stylist. Having read this book, you will be able to ask some basic coloring questions to see if he

knows what he is talking about:

1. What is my natural color level? (Bear in mind that if your regrowth is only about 1/4 inch, there may not be enough hair to determine your natural color. If he's right on, terrific! Even if he's one level off give him the benefit of the doubt. His judgement may have been affected by the lighting in the salon.)

2. What color would you make me if I gave you a free hand? (If he says the sky's the limit, beware. You might also try holding back your formula and asking the stylist what color he would use to achieve your target color. If he's wide of the mark, go somewhere else.)

You may wonder why you need to ask these questions of a professional hairdresser. The answer, sadly, is that many hairdressers know very little about hair color. Consequently, they make the same kind of elementary mistakes that the uninformed home colorist can make. Having read this book there's a strong likelihood that you'll know more about hair color than some of the hairdressers you might encounter.

It's important that you learn to identify a good hairdresser because there will likely be times when you're going to have to place yourself in professional hands whether you want to or not. Here are some of the things that only your hairdresser can do for you.

BLEACHING

Although I have outlined in great detail how to bleach at home, I have done so only because there are products on the market that enable you to do this. However, I strongly advise you not to bleach at home. Go to a technician in a salon. Having read the chapter on bleaching, you will understand not only how precise the application must be, but also how accurately you must judge when to remove the bleach and apply the toner. Bleaching is the most potentially damaging thing you can do to your hair. Therefore, I recommend that you leave it in the hands of someone who knows and understands the process.

COLOR CORRECTION

Many of you will have been coloring your own hair for years. But all of a sudden you may decide that you want to change or improve your color. You cannot do this by yourself at home. All of the techniques I have described in this book are based on the fact that you have not colored your hair before. Color correction — changing from one tint to another — should only be done by your hairdresser.

RETURNING TO YOUR NATURAL COLOR FROM ARTIFICIAL BLONDE

What if you get tired of your bottled blonde hair and decide that you want to return to your natural color? Do not attempt this extremely difficult process at home. It's much more complicated than it might seem. Most clients like to continue to add blonde highlights after they have grown out their color (the technique that I prefer). Most have not remembered themselves as dark as they actually are and the highlights create a much softer and prettier effect than their natural color.

You can also ask your technician to tint the whole head back to the natural color. Still, we must be very careful because, as you will remember, most of natural pigments have been stripped out of the hair in the lightening process. Therefore, before we can change tinted blonde hair back to brown, we will need to put these pigments back. We will not need to bother with the blue or green pigments as there will be enough of these in the brown color that is applied to the hair. But we do need to add orange and red pigments. This process is called **pre-pigmentation.**

Some hairdressers will make their target color and then add about half as much correct pigment (in this case orange or red), and apply this mixture to the hair. Others may apply orange or red pigment directly on the blonde hair and then, after that color has oxidized, apply the brown color. I even remember a hairdresser in California who used henna to pre-pigment the hair and then tinted on top of that. This was a very serious mistake. As the henna washed out the client was left with the brown which hadn't oxidized. Within two weeks her hair was a muddy looking khaki color, and there was nothing that could be done to improve the color because her hair had been hennaed first.

RETURNING TO GRAY

One of the most common question I'm asked is how to return to natural gray after you've been coloring your hair. Quite frankly, I'm usually surprised when a client expresses this desire and yet I can see often there are valid reasons for it. Perhaps you've reached a point in your life where you feel that you want to grow old with the appearance of dignity that gray hair can convey, or you may have become bored with your color. Even more signficantly, you simply may feel that you don't have the time to devote to coloring your hair. You may also have developed an allergy to hair color.

Unfortunately, there is no easy and absolutely "painless" way to return to gray other than letting the color grow out completely. However, a hairdresser can provide an alternative.

For starters, I usually recommend that you grow your hair to one inch regrowth. Then I put highlights — both lighter and darker blondes and browns — into the gray regrowth. This will soften the demarcation line between the outgrowing color and the gray hair, easing the transition.

In some cases where the tinted color is quite light (level 7 or 8 — light blonde to very light blonde), I can put different tones of brown into the blonde and tones of blondes and browns into the gray to further ease the transition.

I have often found that when clients see how gray their hair is as it is growing in, they realize that they do want some of their original color left, and so they will continue with highlights.

The other way to blend in gray hair with an outgrowing tint is to use a semipermanent color. This is applied all over the head, but it will, in fact, only have a positive coloring effect on the gray hair. In my experience, however, the highlighting method is more popular and effective because it requires a visit to the hairdresser only every two to three months, as opposed to every twelve shampoos.

COLOR + PERMANENT WAVE

Both of these processes increase the porosity of your hair. Therefore, if you have a permanent wave on your hair you should not apply permanent color or bleach at home. And if your hair has been bleached or tinted, you should not give yourself a permanent wave at home. You will very likely end up with severely damaged hair.

Both of these processes involve using very strong chemicals on the hair. The permanent wave will break down and restructure the physical shape of each hair. The permanent color or bleach will reorganize or remove the color pigments of the hair through oxidation. Even in the salon there are many situations in which we will recommend that a client not perm her hair if it is permanently colored. Whenever we feel that there is a potential risk, we will always err on the side of caution.

There is another aspect to hair coloring which I have not yet discussed in any detail and that is creative hair coloring. This is the part of the job that color technicians enjoy most. This is where we make our contribution to furthering the art of hairdressing. The following chapter outlines some of these basic techniques and indicates where they are likely to take us in the future.

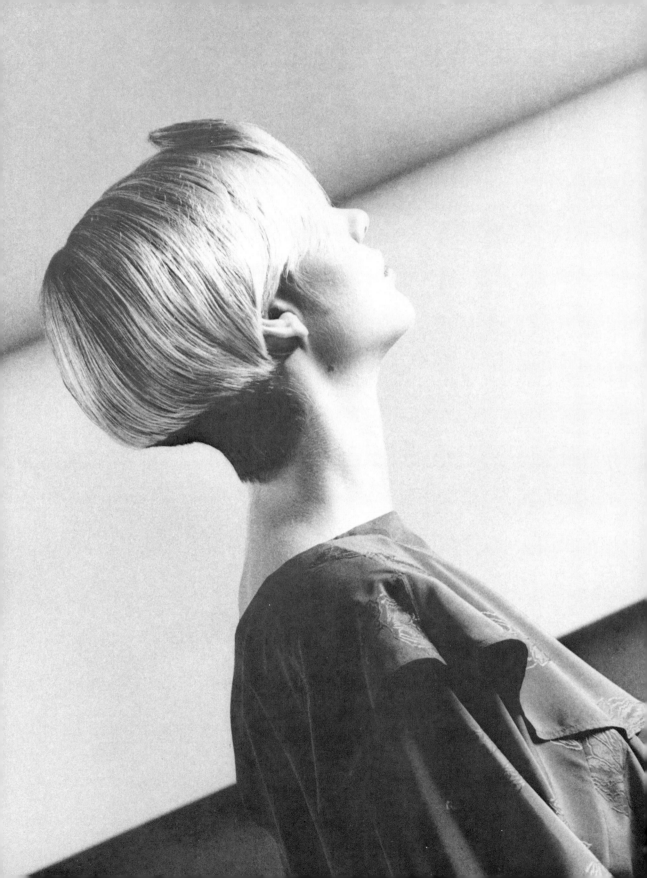

WATERS' COLORS AND THE WAY AHEAD

WATERS' COLORS AND THE WAY AHEAD

WATERS' COLORS WITH A COMB; WATERS' COLORS WITH A BRUSH. FUN THINGS TO DO WITH YOUR HAIR USING TEMPORARY AND SEMIPERMANENT COLORS. THE WAY AHEAD.

In one of the earlier chapters of this book, I gave you some statistics that suggested that between 1955 and 1980, the number of women who went to a hairdressing salon specifically for the purpose of having their hair colored declined from 70 percent to 35 percent. These figures are giving hairdressers a message, and it's one that we shouldn't ignore. Hairdressing has moved with the times, releasing hair from rollers, lacquer and so on. Today women go to the hairdresser specially to have their hair cut.   What are these women telling us? My own feeling is that they're saying that they are not interested in having their hair colored as it was in the past.

There are a number of easily apparent reasons for this. They don't want "roots" and they don't want to see the condition of their hair deteriorate from repeated applications of chemicals. They don't have the time to spend at least an hour and a half at the hairdresser every month. They are also telling us that they resent the fact that hair coloring has become vastly more expensive in the past twenty years, but they have seen an improvement neither in the technique used nor, in many cases, the conditon of their hair. In other words, hairdressing may have kept up with the times, but women don't think they're getting their money's worth when it comes to color.

I'm inclined to feel that often they're right. And yet, in the more innovative salons we have begun to see this situation change, particularly in the last five years. In the world's major cities, women have started to have their hair colored more in salons and this has coincided with a fresh approach to hair color.

At last we began to hear what clients were telling us. They did not want their hair to be solidly colored with one color. Not only did they want some excitement, they were also looking for more natural effects.

As with everything, it seems, when the time is right things do change. It was Vidal Sassoon who was directly responsible for freeing hair in the early Sixties. In late 1976, it was also his artistic team in London that came up with another innovation — that of coloring specific areas of the hair so that the cut and shape of the hair cut would be emphasized.

I was part of that team and during my five years with the Vidal Sassoon organization, I was encouraged to develop these initial ideas further, thereby increasing my own knowledge about the effect of light and shadow on hair. I studied the Impressionist and Postimpressionist painters, reading everything I could find on their own quest to understand the nature of light. This knowledge of how light moves and reflects from an object has given us the masterpieces of, for instance, Renoir, Cezanne and Seurat.

The first technique that was developed at Sassoon's in those early days was their now-famous "Flying Colors." Quite simply, three different colors were separately combed into the hair to emphasize the wave movement in the hairstyle: dark ash which represented shadow; light ash which represented the highest point of light; and a medium warmer color which represented the total color effect. (Because it was warm, the hair would have looked like a total chestnut color.) The result was three-dimensional color in the hair which created much more interest in the hair cut. It also created a much more exciting color for the client.

The success of this very fast (it only took thirty minutes), inexpensive technique, was phenomenal. It seemed that at least 70 percent of our clients who had not had color before couldn't wait. They would go home and talk to their friends who would notice how interesting their hair color was. Then they would want flying colors too.

It was very exciting to be in an atmosphere where instead of simply applying tint to hair, color technicians were looking at different hair shapes and painting colors on the hair to enhance the cut.

We had suddenly become "artists," taking the first step in the direction of how we should be coloring hair.

WATERS' COLORS WITH A COMB

A much simpler version of Flying Colors can be done at home to emphasize the hair around your hairline. To do this, you will need three different permanent hair colors:

one that will lighten your natural color by two levels
one that will darken your natural color by two levels
one that will brighten your natural color by two tones.

Consult the color chart on page 26. It will help you choose the appropriate colors. They will form a triangle on the chart. If, for instance, your natural color is light brown (level 4), your lighter target levels is medium blonde (level 6 in the neutral tones). Therefore, you will use a very light blonde tint (level 8) to achieve this (see page 33). Your darker target level is dark brown (level 2). The warm tone that will brighten your natural color is light warm chestnut brown (level 4).

What You Need

3 different permanent hair colors (see above)
wide-tooth comb
petroleum jelly
gloves
3 non-metallic dishes

To Prepare

1. At least 48 hours before coloring your hair, give yourself a sensitivity test (see page 41). You will not need to do a strand test. If you follow the instructions, you can't go wrong.

2. Mix two capfuls of the darkest color with an equal amount of peroxide in the first dish.

3. Mix two capfuls of the lightest color with an equal amount of peroxide in the second dish.

4. Mix two capfuls of the warm color with an equal amount of peroxide in the third dish. You now have the three colors in separate dishes.

5. Smear petroleum jelly around your hairline.

6. Put on your gloves.

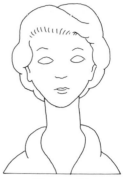

Figure 45

To Color

1. Look in the mirror at the hair nearest your hairline. You will notice that this area is in shadow. Therefore, this is the area that we will emphasize with the darkest color (Figure 45).

2. Dip your wide-tooth comb into the darkest color so that you have color on the first four teeth of the comb.

3. Comb that color gently into the first third of the hair that is nearest the scalp (Figure 46). This will intensify the natural shadow.

4. Wash your comb free of color.

5. Look at your hair again and you will notice that beyond the colored shadow is the color that reflects your true natural color. This is where we are going to place the warmer color. Dip your comb into the warm color, again ensuring that it covers

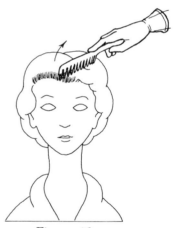

Figure 46

the first four teeth of the comb. Comb the warm color, beginning from the dark color, until you reach the area on your hair that seems to be reflecting a bar of light (Figure 47).

6. Rinse the comb free of color.

7. Dip the comb into the lightest color. Comb it through the area on your hair that is reflecting the light (Figure 48).

8. Allow the colors to develop for 30 minutes.

9. Shampoo your hair.

That's all you need to do. You have not made a dramatic change and yet you will notice that you have added interest to the front of your hair. These subtle applications of color will emphasize the shape of your hair as it moves. People will notice your hair.

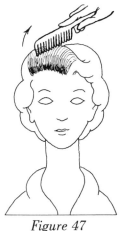

Figure 47

While I was working at Sassoon's in London, I was greatly encouraged to develop my own experiments in how light affects a colored object. About this time, I began to read the work of a turn-of-the-century American physicist, Ogden Rood, whose experiments had greatly influenced the Postimpressionist painters, particularly Georges Seurat. By studying the work of these two men, I learned about the importance of complementary colors. I also began to understand how we could use complementary colors to emphasize subtle changes in hair.

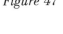

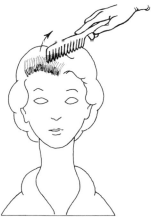

Figure 48

The first result of my experiments was a technique which Sassoon's christened "spotlighting." Spotlighting meant that we could take your shining brown hair a step beyond. We could make it shimmer.

Here's how it works. You'll remember that brown is a tertiary color, which means that all shades of brown result from any combination of the secondary colors (orange, violet and green). Seurat was fascinated by the idea that if you paint a tiny dot of red beside a tiny dot of blue, the eye will optically blend these two colors and see violet. He felt that if he arranged the six primary and secondary colors in certain ways, he could create a shimmering effect of light.

It was reasonable of Seurat to assume that he could achieve this effect, because colors have different wavelengths and will, therefore, meet the eye at different times. Hence, the movement implied in a shimmer. However, the further you stand away from Seurat's paintings, the more gray they appear. A yellow dot and a blue dot do, in fact, combine in the eye to create a positive green. But the greater the distance between the observer and the object, the greater the influence of the white light between them. Eventually it weakens the effect to a grayish green.

Once I understood how this dot technique worked, I realized that these principles could be applied to coloring hair. Secondary colors could be arranged on the hair in tiny dots. By the time they reached the eye of the observer, they would create a shimmer of brown.

WATERS' COLORS WITH A BRUSH

Here is a simplified version of this technique for you to try at home. However, your hair must be short, straight and layered. This may be a beautiful cut, but very little is happening with your hair in terms of movement. The spotlight color will create a unique interest in your hair.

As with Flying Colors, you will need three different permanent colors to spotlight your hair. Consult the color chart on page 26 to help you choose the appropriate colors. If, for example, your hair is light brown (level 4), you will need a dark ash brown tint (level 2 — two levels darker than your natural color); medium ash blonde (level 6 — to achieve this you will need to use a level 8 color, very light ash blonde); and a warm color in

the orange tones at your natural level (light golden chestnut brown — level 4).

What You Need

3 different permanent hair colors (see above)

3 non-metallic dishes

small vent brush
(available at any hair salon — Figure 49)

plastic gloves

petroleum jelly

To Prepare

1. At least 48 hours before coloring your hair, give yourself a sensitivity test (see page 41). You will not need to do a strand test. If you follow these instructions, you can't go wrong.

2. Mix two capfuls of the darkest color with an equal amount of peroxide in the first dish.

3. Mix two capfuls of the lightest color with an equal amount of peroxide in the second dish.

4. Mix two capfuls of the orange color with an equal amount of peroxide in the third dish. You now have three different colors in three separate dishes. (Note: You are only going to color the surface of your hair.)

5. Smear petroleum jelly around your hairline.

6. Put on your gloves.

To Color

1. Gently dip the bristles of the brush into the dark color and shake off the excess color.

2. Looking at your hair in the mirror, decide which

Figure 49

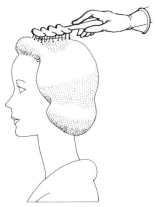

Figure 50

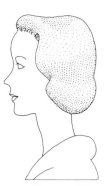

Figure 51

are the areas of shadow over the different parts of the hair you can see. Touch the surface of these parts of the hair with the colored bristles to leave tiny dots of color on your hair (Figure 50).

3. Repeating the procedure, continue to color all the shadows you can see with the darkest color.

4. Rinse the brush free of the dark color.

5. Now look at the areas reflecting your natural warm tones and dip the brush into the orange color. Apply this color to those areas of your hair in the same manner as above. There will be different angles and different shapes of light reflecting on your hair, which will cross through the areas already colored. This is where we will place the lightest color.

6. Dip your brush into the lightest color and apply it to those areas on your hair that are reflecting light. Do not worry if this color overlaps into the other color. It should, as light is never stationary (Figure 51).

7. Allow color to develop for 30 minutes.

8. Shampoo your hair.

One of the great joys of working for Vidal Sassoon in London was that they never allowed you to rest on your laurels. You were constantly stretching your creative mind. The most important influence on me in that respect was Anne Humphries, the head of color and technical research for the Vidal Sassoon organization. She has probably trained more excellent color technicians than anyone else in the world. Certainly I feel very grateful for the help and encouragement she gave me.

At that time, there was a very important exhibition of Postimpressionist paintings in

London. By studying the paintings in great detail, I was able to figure out many of the artists' techniques and adapt them to hair color to emphasize the new shapes that were being created by the stylists.

One great influence was Cezanne whose achievement was to bring the eye of the observer into the distance of his pictures. By leaving patches of white empty on the canvas, he caught the viewer's eye in such a way that it was not only drawn to those spots, but almost wanted to go beyond them. I experimented with this idea in the salon by using bars of horizontal color on the hair. But the technique really wasn't working, so I shelved it temporarily.

A few months later I was living in Canada. It was my first autumn in North America and I was quite overcome by the magnificence of the changing leaves. Suddenly I remembered Cezanne, and I immediately knew what to do. By isolating the hair in foil, I could place thin bars of red, orange and gold throughout the whole head. Unlike highlights, which are vertical, these would move across the head, to create a total movement and blending of different red tones.

Sometime after moving to Canada, I returned to London to participate in an annual international hair show sponsored by *Hairdresser's Journal*. While I was giving seminars and talking about my personal philosophy of hair color, I was challenged by a member of the audience. He informed me that while all these techniques were wonderful, none would work on one-length bobbed hair.

This was like waving a red flag in front of a bull. I turned for inspiration to Monet's paintings of lilies, and there in the effect of wind or a breeze on the water was my answer. Wind makes a glass-like lake shimmer with reflecting tones. When it is healthy, bobbed hair reflects light in a similar way.

Herein lies the source of my technique called "glazing." With three subtle colors very close to the natural one, I color the shapes and shadows of light as it reflects from bobbed hair. The hair is only colored on the surface and the color is applied with a glazing touch from a tint brush. The exciting thing about this effect is that as the wind catches the hair, it disturbs the shape of the hair color. But if the hair is cut well, when the wind drops, the hair will fall into shape and the color will reappear.

FUN THINGS TO DO WITH YOUR HAIR

Basically, the fun things that you can do with your hair fall into two categories:

1. Those that are very temporary, lasting only one shampoo.

2. Those that will last for about three weeks.

Fun with Your Hair Using Temporary Colors

Manufacturers of temporary colors have a range of what we call "party" colors. Basically these are the primary and secondary colors in their purest forms. They can be purchased either through a hairdresser, drugstore or beauty supply shop.

Rule of Thumb: If you are using temporary colors, do a strand test to make sure that your hair is not extremely porous (see Chapter 5). If your hair is very porous, temporary colors will not wash out after one shampoo.

There are also products available that can be sprayed onto the hair to make it gold, silver or black. However, these are extremely pungent, and I advise that you take this into consideration before playing with them. And although they are temporary, they can leave your hair very dry after they are shampooed out.

Glitter dusts can be sprinkled onto your hair. They are available in many colors, including gold and silver.

In most places, although not in every salon, hairdressers can sell you some very bright gel-based temporary colors in shades such as hot pink and emerald green. You can put these on strands of hair wherever you want. Paint a pink stripe down the centre. Go green at the temple. I'm sure that creative minds can come up with some fascinating innovations.

Fun with Your Hair for Three Weeks

The fun things that fall into the more permanent categories should only be done by a color technician. The results are dramatic and you're going to have to live with them for three weeks, so you want to make certain that they're properly done.

You may want to put a very blonde streak in the front of your hair to emphasize a particular area. Since you will only be bleaching a small area, you can have it recolored to your natural color when you get bored with it. This part of your hair will not be in the greatest condition, but it's such a small area that you should be able to live with it.

Although I realize that everybody doesn't want to look like a punk, they have had some innovative ideas in terms of hair coloring. Some of these can certainly be used to a lesser degree on many people's hair for fun.

For instance, there is now a wide range of semipermanent colors available in a myriad of vivid shades such as apricot, aquamarine and scarlet red. They can be used on pre-bleached hair to create the desired color, or they can be applied to natural colors to give a highlighting effect.

If your hair is dark brown, these semipermanent colors will not have much effect, except for the aubergine, dark blue or dark green color which can all add highlights. But if you want a brighter, more dramatic effect, the temporary versions of these colors can be used almost like paint. The other alternative, which is a technique that hairdressers use quite often, is to pre-lighten and then color with one of these semipermanent crayon colors.

THE WAY AHEAD

I hope that armed with all your new knowledge you will now begin to enjoy the excitement of hair color. Better still, I hope that you will encourage your own technician to come up wth some creative solutions of his or her own. If this book starts you or your hairdresser thinking in new ways about color, then I will have accomplished what I set out to do.

This, of course, is only the first step. The second lies with the manufacturers who must experiment with their products to give the technicians the kinds of raw materials we need. We are all looking for a new type of hair coloring product that will not damage the hair at all, and yet will produce all the coloring effects that permanent color gives us now.

Moreover, as professionals, we need to increase our knowledge of how we can use color to produce more natural results without solidly coloring the hair. Maybe what we have done with this book is to create the perfect triad of knowledge. Not only do the manufacturers and the hairdressers know about color, you, the client, now has access to much of that information. This allows you to influence the direction that you want your own hair color to take. That, I think, is the way ahead.

GLOSSARY

Ammonia: A liquid gas. It ignites hydrogen peroxide to create oxidation, which takes place during all permanent coloring and bleaching processes.

Bleaching: A process that strips all pigment from the hair. It must take place during all dramatic lightening processes. Also called stripping.

Conditioner: A creamy softening agent that allows easy combing of hair after shampooing. Another term for a cream rinse.

Cortex: The inside of the hair which contains all the protein and natural color.

Cuticle: The outside layer of the hair. The cuticle forms a protection for the cortex.

Henna: A permanent natural hair color that does not use oxidation to color the hair.

Highlifting tint: Permanent hair color that will lighten hair more than four levels of the natural color. It is used to achieve shades of blonde and is only available at a salon.

Highlights: Fine strands which are separated from the main body of hair and lightened with either bleach or tint to a very light blonde.

Hydrogen peroxide: The catalyst which, when combined with ammonia, produces oxidation.

Lowlights: Fine strands which are separated from the main body of hair and tinted tones of brown or red.

Melanin: A natural chemical of the body which is the source of color for the hair and the skin.

Moisturizer: An agent for dry hair which adds moisture in the form of protein.

Natural color: The color that grows naturally in the hair.

Natural color level: The numerical degree of darkness or lightness of your natural color, according to a color chart.

Oxidation: The process that occurs when hydrogen peroxide combines with ammonia. It softens and swells the hair, generating heat, and permits a change in the natural hair color by either tinting or bleaching.

Partings: The small separations of hair to which color is applied.

Permanent color: Also know as a tint. When mixed with hydrogen peroxide and ammonia it oxidizes in the cortex to permanently change the natural color pigment of the hair.

Pigment: Tiny molecules of color found in the cortex of the hair.

Porosity: The ability of the hair to absorb and retain a color.

Powder bleach: A bleach in powder form. It is used in salons exclusively for highlights. It should not be used on the scalp.

Protein pack treatment: Intensive protein treatment which fills the hair with all the necessary proteins. The frequency of use depends upon the condition of the hair.

Rinse: Another term for a semipermanent color.

Sections: The four quarters hair is separated into to create an uncluttered area so that color can be applied neatly to the partings.

Semipermanent color: A color that lies on and inside the cuticle of the hair. It will last for six to fourteen shampoos, depending upon the type of product used.

Sensitivity test: A test to make sure that you are not allergic to hair color.

Strand test: A test to determine the natural color of the hair. It is also used to test hair-coloring products to ensure that they will produce the proper target color.

Temporary color: It lies on the cuticle of the hair and will usually only last for one shampoo.

Tint: A hairdresser's term for a permanent color.

Tinting: The process of coloring the hair with permanent color.

Tone: The secondary hair color that appears throughout one's natural or neutral hair color.

Toner: A semipermanent color that is applied to pre-bleached hair, giving it pastel blonde tones.

Virgin hair: Hair that has not been chemically changed in either structure, as in permanent waving, or in color, as in bleaching or tinting.

CREDITS

All hair color by Peter Waters
unless otherwise credited.

Cover Model: Ann Spence
Judy Welch Model Agency
Hair: Ian Djurkin
Make-up: Gordon Espinet

2 Model: Ann Spence
Jucy Welch Model Agency
Hair: Velda
Make-up: Gordon Espinet
Clothes: Metropolis

14 Model: Andrea Des Roches
Judy Welch Model Agency
Hair: Velda
Make-up: Gordon Espinet
Clothes: Eve et Lui

19 Model: Jane Ashley
Nexus Personal Management
Hair: Bryan Prefer
Make-up: Lucienne Zammit
Necklace: De Val Jewellers,
Toronto
Earrings: Beni Sung, Toronto

22 Model: Frencesca D'Addario
Judy Welch Model Agency
Hair: Ian Djurkin
Make-up: Gordon Espinet

28 Model: Laura Francis
Fulcher's Line
Hair: Velda
Make-up: Lucienne Zammit
Clothes: Asta Fashions Ltd.

37 Model: Maggie Borg
Jo Penney
Hair: Ron Fava
Make-up: Lucienne Zammit

38 Model: Peggy Sands
Judy Welch Model Agency
Hair: Ron Fava
Make-up: Gordon Espinet

46 Model: Catherine Howley
Judy Welch Model Agency
Hair: Velda
Make-up: Lucienne Zammit

56 Model: Jayne Lewis
Judy Welch Model Agency
Hair: Ron Fava
Make-up: Lucienne Zammit
Clothes: Asta Fashions Ltd.

68 Model: Maria Zupet
Fulcher's Line
Hair: Michael Kearns
Color: Robert Fleet
Make-up: Gordon Espinet

73 Model: Fauna
Hair: Bryan Prefer
Make-up: Lucienne Zammit
Clothes: Empress Furs Ltd.

74 Model: Bridgete Hunter
Judy Welch Model Agency
Hair: Ron Fava
Make-up: Gordon Espinet

82 Model: Beverly Pearson
Judy Welch Model Agency
Hair: Velda
Make-up: Gordon Espinet
Clothes: Eve et Lui

85 Model: Brenda Gale
Fulcher's Line
Hair: Michael Kearns
Make-up: Gordon Espinet

91 Model: Gabriella Mutone
Fanfare
Hair: Ron Fava
Make-up: Lucienne Zammit

92 Model: Kate Wheeler
Jerry Lodge Model
Management
Hair: Ron Fava
Color: Sean Fleet
Make-up: Gordon Espinet
Clothes: Suit – Marcello
Tarantino
Blouse – Asta Fashions Ltd.

100 Model: Leslee Bond
Sherrida Personal Manage-
ment Inc.
Hair: Ian Djurkin
Make-up: Gordon Espinet

105 Model: Anita Wilson
Fulcher's Line
Hair: Velda
Make-up: Lucienne Zammit

107 Model: Joan Bailey
Jo Penney Inc.
Hair: Ron Fava
Make-up: Gordon Espinet

109 Model: Sandra Marquis
Hair: Ian Djurkin
Make-up: Gordon Espinet
Clothes: Marilyn's

110 Model: Peggy Sands
Judy Welch Model Agency
Hair: Ron Fava
Make-up: Gordon Espinet

116 Model: Linda Werner
Hair: Ron Fava
Make-up: Lucienne Zammit
Clothes: Eve et Lui